Mel Giedroyc was born in Epsom District Hospital in 1968. She looked like a frog and none of the midwives would pick her up. Her first word was 'Leatherhead'. She now lives in London with her husband and two daughters and does her bit in the comedy duo Mel and Sue.

For B, F and V.

In loving memory of E.

from here to maternity

Love and thanks to my editor Andrew Goodfellow for his patience, expertise and expense account. To my friends who kept me going through the blocks, especially Rache, Nem, Tommy, Brian, Cid, Ghiz, Jack, Perce, Ruth, Susie, Anna, Zumbs and Emma K. To Samira, Molly, Lucy and Deborah at ICM for putting up with my rambling. To Caroline Murphy for holding the fort, and John Nettles for his dancing blue eyes. To Dad, Miko, Dodi, Kasia, Philip and Tom for plying me with drink when required, and for making encouraging noises. To Tom M, Ness, Chris, Jo, Mike and Rosemary for taking me into the bosom. To Ben and Mum for being loving yet scarily rigorous proofreaders. Finally to my sister Coky – we squabbled, we feuded, we laughed – her input is always invaluable and I couldn't have written the book without her. Oh, and someone who calls herself Sue Perkins. She keeps phoning me. I have no idea who she is.

MEL GIEDROYC

from here to maternity

EBURY PRESS

1 3 5 7 9 10 8 6 4 2

First published 2004 by Ebury Press,
an imprint of Random House,
20 Vauxhall Bridge Road, London SW1V 2SA

Random House Australia (Pty) Limited
20 Alfred Street, Milsons Point, Sydney,
New South Wales 2061, Australia

Random House New Zealand Limited
18 Poland Road, Glenfield, Auckland 10, New Zealand

Random House South Africa (Pty) Limited
Endulini, 5a Jubilee Road, Parktown 2193, South Africa

The Random House Group Limited Reg. No. 954009

www.randomhouse.co.uk

Printed and bound in Great Britain by Mackays of Chatham plc, Kent

A CIP catalogue record for this book is available from the British Library.

Cover designed by Jon Gray
Typeset by seagulls

ISBN 0 09188 686 4

Sunday

THERE IS NO DAWN CHORUS in our part of London. It's more of a solo performed by a lone pigeon bemoaning his gnarled feet. This morning I was unfortunate enough to hear it. You see, I didn't sleep very well. Rather tossy and turny. I dreamt I was being chased by a strange man with long, sandy eyelashes. I was in a pair of concrete-filled waders, so I couldn't run away. I woke myself up and couldn't get back to sleep because I kept seeing the sandy eyelashes whenever I shut my eyes. I eventually realised they were mine. Must get them dyed.

Some might say that I am obsessed with sleep. Before I retire each night I like to work out how many hours I'm going to get. If it's between ten and twelve, I'm positively gleeful and jump into my bed like a toddler into a puddle. If it's in the eight- to ten-hour ballpark I am serene, verging on smug. Pulling back the covers, I'll give them a little pat and head for nod with a self-satisfied smile, like somebody at a classical concert who hums along to the music. If I know I'm getting less than eight, I'm resentful. Fewer than six and I consider putting in a morning call to Amnesty International. It's quite simply inhumane.

For as long as I can remember I have slept like a baby – seriously deep, Sleeping Beauty-type slumber. Of course, I don't for a second mean that I *look* like Sleeping Beauty when I'm out – a chloroformed chipmunk would be more accurate.

I take after my Lithuanian dad's side of the family – the hardy Baltic ability to hunker down and sleep any time, any place. I have slept standing up. I have slept in a shower. I have slept under a thin layer of felt. I have slept on gravel, on a bicycle and next to a man pleasuring himself in a sleeping bag. (I was not in the sleeping bag with him, I hasten to add.) I have slept in the dentist's chair undrugged, while the dentist filled a tooth. I have slept in a ferry terminal loo, a cinema foyer and a canoe.

I even managed to grab a few winks onstage in a production of *King Lear*. While Gloucester was having his eyes put out, I was closing mine at the back of the stage. No location is too difficult for me – if there's an equivalent of the Mile High Club for kippers, then get me a membership card. My God, I love to sleep.

So I'm terse today and can't work out why I didn't sleep. Was the temperature wrong in our bedroom? Pretty clement, I'd say. Was Dan nicking the duvet? No more than usual. Had I eaten any cheese just before going to bed? Was it noisy? Who am I trying to kid? I once had a nap at a rave. Curled up for two hours. Right by the speakers.

Monday

I DID ALL MY PREP LAST NIGHT. Went to bed nice and early, around the ten o'clock mark after a relaxing Tension Tamer Tea, safe in the knowledge that I was on for at least nine hours. The previous night's blip had left me feeling nicely tired. Not dog tired, just a comforting ache around the shoulders. Jim-jams on, slippers off, lights out.

I woke up at 2 a.m., then at three, five and half six. A ruddy joke. Restless, bored and shockingly awake, I finally whispered to Dan, 'Are you asleep?' really loudly so he'd have to wake up. He mumbled, 'Mmm thirsty? Water … go to the loo,' then turned over and immediately made contented, rodent-like snores.

This morning has been rather too long for my liking. Both of us are working at home this week, which can be trying at the best of times. Although Dan's real ambition is to write film scripts, at the moment he is working as a subtitler – translating other people's films from English into French and German. Which makes him a bit of a swot really.

Dan and I met when we were at college, both studying French. I knew instantly it was love when I saw him smoking a Gauloise. So laid-back and sophisticated – sitting on the steps outside the library, his eyes squinting into the middle distance – he could have been in an Ultravox video. True, the impact was lessened by the fact that he was also wearing patchwork trousers and white socks, but still, a filterless French cigarette!

One of the key differences between us since that day is that Dan has actually gone on to make use of his education, while I have forgotten everything I was taught. Recently, in Paris, I couldn't remember what the French was for 'weekend', until Dan, rather smugly, reminded me that the French for 'weekend' is 'le weekend'.

So while Dan's poring over a French dictionary checking the best way to phrase 'The geezer's tooled up ain't he?' for the gangster flick he's working on, I'm pretending to be busy at the kitchen table. I'm supposed to be researching the Male Pill. I'm not a scientist or health worker. In fact I don't do anything remotely useful. I'm a presenter. On radio and TV. I have to come clean and say that work's been a bit slow of late. But hurray! I've been asked to present an item on male contraception in a health show for Bravo cable channel. My brief is to make it 'pithy, wry, amusing, but not smutty'. But at the moment I feel about as pithy as a very old orange that should be thrown out of the fruit bowl.

Dan's work is obviously going very well. He keeps repeating French phrases out loud to himself and laughing. Feeling tired and sorry for myself, I ask Dan for some help, but his only comment is 'The Male Pill? Make it lager-flavoured and it might catch on!'

Tuesday

Tonight I brought out the big gun: the Virgin Airways long-haul sleeping mask. It had worked a treat for the row of nuns behind me on the New York flight a few years back – each sister blissfully slumped with 'Virgin' emblazoned across her crumpled brow as they snored in holy unison over the Atlantic.

Nothing. It blocked out the light, but still didn't take me anywhere near the shadowy forests of Lethe. Not even halfway. I probably got as far as Leatherhead in sleep terms.

It's three in the morning. I'm normally into my second round of REMs by now. The irony is I'm writing this by the light of Dan's special reading glasses that *he* normally uses, so as not to disturb *me*. DJs use them, they're like plastic sunglasses with a light on each corner of the lens – a kind of ravey Davy lamp. I don't think Sleeping Beauty modelled these either.

I try to wake Dan up by focusing the beams of light directly into his face. I then do a quick impression of the Underworld DJ who wore them at Glastonbury in 1997 and I sing 'Lager lager lager!' into Dan's ear. No response. I then whisper too loudly that I'm bored and does he fancy a quick game of Boggle? His response, with little movement, is 'Bugger Boggle' closely followed by '… and Bugger off'. He's turned over again into his sleep and is soon chomping contentedly on some imaginary titbit.

I'd once read somewhere (laughingly and a little smugly – 'Insomnia? Me? Ha!') that if you can't sleep you should get up, strip and remake your bed very carefully and energetically, to hospital standards. I briefly toy with the idea of just stripping to see if that'll wake Dan up, but feel loath to undock myself from my beloved pyjamas. I'll go for bed-stripping. I leap out of bed, do a couple of star-jumps at its foot, touch my toes several times with some little 'hrrumphs', then jog round to Dan's side and start to strip the bed. Crick his head round, slip the pillow out from underneath him. Lovely. Pillowcase off, humming as I go. Whip off the duvet and try to grab the bottom sheet. Everything carried out quickly and clinically. Dan opens one eye slowly. He is not amused.

'Oh. You're awake!' I say brightly. 'Can't you sleep either, love?'

'Of course I can't bloody sleep if you take the bloody duvet away. What the hell are you doing?'

'Just stripping and remaking the bed. You might have to get up actually so I can get a proper purchase on this bottom sheet.'

At which Dan gets up and leaves the room. I hear him shuffle downstairs and the living-room door slams behind him. Oops.

I try to carry on regardless. But changing a duvet is a hard enough act of domestic engineering in the cold light of day. My actions suddenly appear as pointless and ridiculous as indeed they actually are. What the hell am I doing? It's three in the morning. I take the executive decision to go downstairs and snuggle up with Dan on the sofa. Not a lot of room or sympathy down there, but I'll make it into an affectionate gesture. I scrape plaintively on the living-room door like a sad little gerbil.

'Dan! Can I come and lie with you?'

Wednesday

DAN PUT IN A VERY comfortable nine-hour shift on the sofa under a travel rug. I slept for half an hour folded up by the bookshelf. Whenever I valiantly tried to snuggle up beside him, he propelled me from the sofa by poking me. He finally sat bolt upright and threatened to divorce me if I even thought about trying to wake him up again. I thought I'd best leave it. I watched a bit of Open University with the sound down. Even that failed to send me to sleep.

What if this is it? What if I've gone over to the other side and become an insomniac? I'll turn into the undead, a walking zombie with eye bags, grey hair and a constant bad taste in my mouth. My brain will go to seed, I'll lose my job and be stretchered away, laughing and dribbling. I'm panicked by the thought. Without sleep I will be a husk.

Another Wednesday

One sleepless week on. Went out today with Dan to look for a new car. Our old one has recently started to sound like a tug boat. People openly swear at us in the street now when we drive past because it makes such a terrible noise.

Dan knows a hell of a lot about cars – he openly admits to watching *Top Gear* and enjoying it – and has had his nose in *Auto Trader* for much of the last week. For him, this is an exciting adventure. I am humourless about the whole car purchase issue and have my own particular ideas. I don't want a neat little baby that holds the road at 70 mph or any of that malarkey. I just want one that matches my wardrobe, has a working hazard triangle and a nice clean set of ashtrays.

The car we're going to see is up the A40. Dan is hale and chatty, shouting above the headache-inducing clatter that is our car. I look like a cadaver in the passenger seat, pale as a goth and terse as a newsreader. The more Dan talks about the relative pros and cons between a four- and six-cylinder engine, the more I want to barf. And then the car starts to splutter. Splutter, stutter, splatter and finally drone and conk. And there we are on the side of the A40 with ten thousand tons of juggernaut rumbling perilously past our trousers. Dan loves a challenge like this – and scrambles underneath the car quicker than a bridesmaid under a wedding table. Left on my own, I'm suddenly overwhelmed by the need to get on all fours on the grassy verge and puke like some sort of large cat. I haven't had travel-sickness like this since I was a kid.

Dan's doing his best under the car and we hear the distant wail of several ambulances and police cars. It's always depressing to hear that sound on a motorway. There must be a pile-up somewhere; I hope nobody's dead. I do a little sign of the cross. It's only when the wailing is so loud that I can't hear myself think, and a very jolly paramedic in a pea-green boiler suit is talking urgently into my face that I realise that the cavalcade of emergency vehicles has arrived for us.

Somebody phoned from a mobile saying they saw a woman on all fours in distress and a man dead underneath an old BMW. Are we all right? Do we need any help? How mortifying. Even worse, I feel my eyes are starting to brim with tears as I talk to the paramedic – she's so strong and comforting. Once they've left, I wipe my tears and the AA arrive. Again the brimming starts – I feel so emotional about all these amazing people in uniform being such towers of strength and calm. Keith tows us all the way home. I can smell sick in my nostrils and my humour barrels are pretty much scraped. Dan is clenching and de-clenching his teeth, which makes his jawline wiggle – never a good sign. It's because every other person in a car that passes looks at our lame-arse car on the end of the tow-rope and laughs.

Thursday

DAN'S GONE OUT on his own to buy us a second-hand car, with strict and technical instructions from me – 'Make it cool, groovy and kind of laid-back retro.' I feel too rough to go with him, and frankly I'm relieved. I don't want to stand around kicking tyres, trying to sound interested in the workings of a fuel-injected, turbo-diesel 3.8-litre hatchback, or whatever. Anyway, I'm supposed to be at home finishing my male pill research. After a brief dalliance at my computer, I'm on the sofa watching one of those daytime TV confessional programmes. Today's theme is 'My fella can't stop clowning around', and it is Louise and her boyfriend Pete's turn to receive the sympathetic attentions of the host. Pete literally is a circus clown and is sitting there in the studio complete with red nose, silly wig and sinister flapping shoes. Louise really loves Pete but is threatening to leave him if he doesn't start taking something – anything – seriously. But he is always making gags, gurning, tooting on his horn and falling over. Louise is sick of it and wants him to start acting like the fifty-year-old that he is.

'It's so frustrating, Pete and I will go to a Parents' Evening and he'll just make jokes to the teachers. Once he even sprayed one with a plastic flower. It was sad. Nobody thought it was at all funny.'

While Louise is saying this, Pete is up and clowning around in front of the studio audience, doing a silly walk and making faces behind Louise's back.

'You see? He's doing it now. Honestly, I just can't cope.'

Poor Louise. The thing is – it is funny. The audience are starting to giggle and I am too. The more thunderous Louise's expression becomes, the more hilarious Pete's antics seem. I start to laugh, and then tears start to mix with the laughter. Then suddenly I am crying. It goes on for a good couple of minutes before I get a grip of myself. I really don't know what is happening to me. Is this the start of some kind of breakdown? I feel panicked and out of control and decide there and then, as I wipe the tears and snot away with a tea towel, to pay a visit to Dr Sweeting.

'Do you need to see the doctor or the nurse this time?'

My regular bouts of hypochondria have made me something of a favourite at the local surgery.

'Well, I brimmed at a paramedic and have just cried at a clown.'

'Fine. Ten-thirty with Doctor Sweeting on Thursday all right for you?'

Friday

My mum doesn't believe in the existence of stress. I've just phoned her for some sympathy. I tell her I'm not sleeping and that I think it could be stress related.

'Stress didn't really exist when I was your age. Why don't you go and do some ironing? Or weed the flowerbeds for some fresh air? All of you younger generation have got nothing to put up with, yet you seem to go down like ninepins with these imaginary complaints. You've got mobile phones and kitchen appliances coming out of your ears, but half of you lot are on those happy pills.'

I adore my mother but sometimes she gets the wrong end of the stick. That's what mothers are for, I guess – if she was getting the right end of the stick that would be my end of the stick, and we wouldn't both be able to hold it. I like us tussling with the stick – it makes life much more interesting. She does have a point though – what the hell do I have to be stressed about? I have Dan, we make ends meet, we have a home and we're both healthy. Maybe I'm stressed because there's nothing to be stressed about – Heaven Syndrome or whatever it's called.

Saturday

DAN HAS FINALLY TURNED UP trumps in the hunt for a new car. This morning he blindfolded me and led me out into the street. When he whipped off the headscarf, I practically fainted. It is a vision of retro-grooviness: a pistachio-green soft-top two-seater with faux leather interior and cream hub-caps, and it's called a Rigoletto! It's a bit ragged round the edges but who cares? It's a tad pretentious but so what? We are a freelance London media couple in our early thirties: it's our duty to be pretentious. We are flying the flag for all thirty-somethings who like to think they're ten years younger than they really are, whose Habitat bread-bins are chocka with ciabatta, who put piles of shells on their stairs and hang a hippy hammock from their year off in Kathmandu in their pretend-messy backyards.

For the first time in days I'm lifted. I nip upstairs to don a bit of slap. Dan puts on his mirrored shades, which always make me wince – they're those purple-petrolly ones that cricketers wear. We jump in the front, all smiles, and start her up. We test-drive the stereo too with *The Best 80s Album in the World Ever!* for that final touch of Ironic Retro. We sing along to Heaven 17's 'Temptation' with shameless verve as we scoot down the road in our very own lifestyle ad.

We park conspicuously outside the Pelican pub and I grab a table outside while Dan goes to the bar. We nurse our drinks, read the papers and gaze occasionally in loving reverie at our hip new urban chariot. Until, while Dan's at the loo, I am rudely awakened by an unwelcome debate at the table next to us.

They had arrived shortly after we did and look either like students, or they could be doing their GCSEs for all I know. I find it hard to tell these days.

'It's one of those twat-mobiles.'

'They sell for a mint to sad middle-aged tossers who think it makes them look cool and cutting edge.'

'Talk about the emperor's new clothes. It's one step up from a three-wheeler spazzer car.'

'They're so light they can get blown over in high winds. Some mates of mine once lifted one out of its parking space and hid it round the corner. Fucking hilarious.'

I'm very quickly a deep shade of red. If Dan could hear what's being said he'd want to reverse over them.

'A fiver says the driver's over forty, wearing wanky sunglasses and suffers from erectile dysfunction.'

My heart is beating fast, my whole body buzzing with shame and indignation. 'Twat' I can deal with. 'Sad' I can accept. But 'middle-aged'? That hurt.

They have no idea we are the owners and I'd like to keep it that way. Let's hope they're not here for a session and move on swiftly. I'd like to leave as soon as we have the opportunity.

Dan wanders back, oblivious to his erectile dysfunction problem.

'Come on, let's go.'

'Fancy another spin?' He smiles with modest pride.

'Er … perhaps a walk first?'

Dan looks confused as I snatch his shades from his head and drop them in my bag, snapping it shut.

We walk for an hour and, thank God, they've left the table. I leap into our emotionally tarnished vehicle and Dan starts her up. He can't understand why I spend the entire journey home hunched over in the brace position.

Sunday

THE DAY OF REST and still no sleep. I'm now as frazzled as a supply teacher. Is this the start of a mid-life crisis? Am I stressed about middle age? I am thirty-three years old – not getting any younger, granted. I'll also admit I've let my hairstyle go and my wardrobe tends to stop at Fergie's wedding era. There's also a bit too much navy entering it these days, which is a worry. But I still wear trainers! I still listen to groovy music – even if it is more chill-out than nose-bleed trance. And the house is now the place I listen to House music. I can tell you who Grooverider, Blue and Fifty Cent are. I watched *Pop Idol.* And I have never, ever worn a piece of semi-precious jewellery on a silver chain around my neck. A piece of garnet or rose quartz on a chain is pretty much the same as wearing a T-shirt saying Middle-Aged Tosser on it.

Thirty-three years old. The same age as Jesus was when he died and look what he'd achieved! He'd performed miracles, created a major world religion, died and come back to life. What have I achieved? Joined the Dennis the Menace fan club, struggled to Grade Five on the piano, got hooched a lot at college and then worked in daytime TV for a couple of years. What is my philosophy? What would I fight for? Who am I?

Before I start to sound too much like a Tibetan hippy or a question on *Going For Gold* I realise I know exactly who and what I am. I'm a desperate wannabe, H-dropping, spineless, liberal, knowledge-less waffling old bore who's approaching middle age as fast as my quad bike can get me there.

Right. There's going to be some life-topiary going on around here. Snip, snip, snip away my tawdry wardrobe, snip at my dodgy hair, snip at my directionless lifestyle. Leaves are going to be turned.

Just as soon as I get some kip.

Monday

I WAKE UP MID-AFTERNOON having caught a few much-needed hours after another long and sleepless night. My left eye now has a permanent twitch in it like Chief Inspector Dreyfus from the Pink Panther films. My hair is greasy and my mouth tastes like an old grip-bag. I am completely and utterly bereft of humour.

I fill up the kettle, giving the sink a sharp sniff as I do. There's a terrible whiff of asparagus about the place. The phone rings and I grab it.

'Oh hi, gorgeous, it's Mima!'

It's Jemima, my agent. Her voice always sounds like she's just drunk neat bleach.

'Hello, Jemima.'

'Listen, my honey-darling, something really good's just come through. A kind of reality-dating-surveillance show. Twenty eps, for daytime. Are we interested?'

It's at this point of the conversation that I realise my agent has just called me 'my honey-darling'. I can't let that pass and decide to try and outdo her luvvyness with some fluffy terms of endearment of my own.

'Reality-daytime-dating you say? I'll certainly think about it ... hot nuts.'

There is a slight pause.

'Er ... great, love. I'll fax over the treatment for you to have a look at, OK?'

'Brilliant ... dew flaps.' I've got the giggles now.

'Sorry, what was that?'

'I said dew flaps.'

'Oh. Right. OK then, babe. Expect something through on the fax and we'll talk later.'

'OK. Bye-bye ... love-chops.'

Terrible irony deficiency in the media industry. Perhaps you can get supplements for it?

Dan comes in at around six and asks me how I'm feeling. A lot better for some kip is the answer. I mention the acrid smell of asparagus. But Dan can't smell anything and says it's my imagination.

Tuesday

SLEPT LIKE A LOG LAST NIGHT. Thirteen hours! My face looks like a puffa fish and I've got chipolata sausages for eyelids, but hey, at least I feel human again.

The life-pruning starts here. I go straight for a therapeutic wardrobe blitz. Dear me, there's some grim old gubbins in here: a T-shirt with armpit stains, some striped espadrilles, a pair of marble-wash jeans and, the worst offender of the lot, a navy suit. Stick some epaulettes on it and you've got a commanding officer on board HMS *Invincible*. What the hell possessed me to buy that? I tie up the bulging binbag and throw it down the stairs ready to bequeath to Marie Curie. This is all going very well.

Over lunch I read the fax which has come through from my agent, giving me all the gory details about the job offer. It's a new daytime show called *Ex Maniac*. The show is pitched as part *Big Brother*, part *Blind Date* and part *The Ipcress File*. The gist of it seems to be that I would sit in a small hidden booth in a shopping centre in the company of a divorced man or woman. They have to spy on shoppers using hidden surveillance cameras, choose the person most unlike their ex-partner and hilariously ask them for a date. Then they both get a makeover. The project has enough cheese dripping off it to sate a Swiss skier's appetite, but frankly our coffers are running a tad low, and the show would be screened in the morning, so nobody's going to see it. Unless they're in prison.

As I read on I suddenly get a tang of that asparagus again. Only really strongly this time. It lurks around the back of my throat and makes me salivate like I'm just about to be sick. I can see it in my mind's eye – a large spear of asparagus oozing with butter, its nobbly head bowing over and dripping in its own hot, lardy sauce. A shard of vomit founts from between my lips and spatters the fax. I cover my mouth and run to the downstairs loo, which I liberally pebble-dash.

Dan reminds me this evening that the last time either of us ate asparagus was two years ago at a wedding. He's turned into Sherlock Holmes, pacing round the kitchen scratching his chin, determined to get to the bottom of this intriguing asparagus whodunnit.

Wednesday

DAN AND I DECIDE TO TAKE A SPIN in the new car. As we wander outside, I see the Rigoletto in all of its pistachio glory. Then from nowhere I feel the vom rising in my throat. Something about the sight of that car – its colour, shape, everything. I hug a lamp-post and park my throw-up right there in the street. A neighbour rounds the corner with her trolley and crosses to the other side of the street. I attempt a faltering wave in her direction but she just keeps going.

'What is it, love?' says Dan, crouched over the sick like Hercule Poirot and looking as if he is actually about to sift through it with his fingers.

'It's the car!' I say. 'It makes me feel sick.'

Thursday

'THE CAR?' SAYS DR SWEETING.

'Yes, Doctor Sweeting.'

I always like to use the formal title with her. She's a little twig of a woman, always immaculately dressed in a black suit and court shoes, with a face not dissimilar to a young Valerie Singleton.

'Right. And is it like a motion sickness when you're driving around in the car?'

'No, Doctor Sweeting. It is the sight of it parked outside the house.'

'Does it evoke some sort of memory for you?'

'Not really.'

Blank silence.

'I'm also experiencing a strong smell of asparagus lurking around the house, and to be honest, Doctor Sweeting, I think I can smell it as we speak.'

'Right.' She's looking though my notes.

'And I'm absolutely knackered and I've been crying quite a lot. There was a really sweet clown on telly the other morning whose wife didn't understand him—'

'Mel,' she whips out a calendar, 'can I ask you when your last period was?'

Of course! Why the hell didn't I think of it before? This is an almighty dose of PMT. It makes total sense – the crying, the feeling tired. I am so dumb sometimes. How embarrassing to waste a doctor's precious time with this. Still, it's a relief to know there's a rational reason behind all this weirdness.

'Of course. It must have been about ... ooh, about four weeks ago, I think.'

I am suddenly reminded of my sister Kate. When we were growing up she always wrote the letter P down in her diary on the day her period was due. I'd had a crafty sneak in her hessian-bound book where she had earnestly logged things like 'Flute lesson 5 p.m.' and 'CND barbecue, 6–9 p.m.' Then I discovered all these Ps – written in red felt-tip, which I now think was overdoing it. Not only that, midway between the Ps were a whole load of Os in yellow felt-tip.

'What are all those yellow Os, Katie?' I laughed, as she snatched the book away from me.

'It's the days when I ovulate.'

Being ten years old at the time I had no idea what ovulating was, but I thought she was over-egging it. When we were all round the table having supper that night and Dad asked us what we had planned for the next day I announced that I was going to go out roller-skating and Kate was going to ovulate.

'About four weeks ago, you say?'

'Yes. I'm bad about keeping track, Doctor Sweeting. Unlike my sister Kate who used to write P and O in her diary. And she wasn't talking about a ferry trip!'

Dr Sweeting breathes in gently so that her nostrils pinch just ever so slightly. Tiny manoeuvres like this speak volumes with the good doctor. That infinitesimally small gesture from her actually means: 'Shut the bloody hell up, you blithering twannock. I have a list of three thousand patients in this surgery and I really haven't got the time to hear anecdotes about your stupid family.'

'Can I make a suggestion, Mel?'

'That I leave here and stop wasting your time?'

'No. That you go into the toilet and do a pregnancy test.'

'I'm sorry?'

I feel as though someone's placed an astronaut's helmet on my head. Everything sounds and looks slightly fudged and faraway. Dr Sweeting's mouth is moving and she's reaching down into her drawer to give me one of those lolly-stick things to take with me into the loo. She's probably explaining to me how to operate it, then again she might be telling me that she's a big fan of happy-handbag house and has been since the mid-nineties. I really don't know. All I'm hearing in my head is a kind of watery rumble that must be the daily experience of the goldfish. I wander towards the Ladies with my face looking pretty fish-like too. The open-mouthed disbelief of the guppy.

This is only the second time I've done a pregnancy test kit. The first time I was sixteen years old. I'd stayed over at my schoolfriend Lucy's house on a Saturday night. Her parents were away and being the kind of mule-wearing, workshop-everything-through-with-your-kids type of parents they were, they'd allowed us to 'look after' the house while they were away. We'd thrown a bit of a goth soirée for us, our mate Rach and two gawky boys, whom we knew very slightly. Their hair was back-combed and they wore overcoats from Oxfam. The mood was cool and non-committal and the soundtrack was very much The Cure. We'd met up with the gawksters earlier in the evening at Martyr's Memorial, which involved sitting on its stone steps and looking as if we were above it all and possibly considering suicide. It was terrible for piles.

A few glasses of our favourite tipple, the Purple Parachute – three parts cider to two parts blackcurrant to one part Schnapps – had a very quick and violent effect. The next thing I remember was waking up in the morning on the sofa with one of the goth's spikes of hard, sugared hair sticking into my eye. I had the vaguest memories of kissing him quite a lot and that it had tasted of smoky bacon crisps. Nothing else could feasibly have happened. He still had his overcoat on, for goodness' sake and I was fully clothed. I felt awful. I got home later that day hung-over and starving. I couldn't help myself from wolfing loads of snacks, which basically convinced my teenage logic that I must be pregnant. What's the first thing you do when you're up the stick? Eat loads. There you go, all the evidence I needed. I couldn't sleep that night for the torment of it. Mum and Dad would be terribly ashamed of their youngest daughter's fall from grace. I would be forced to run away to the countryside like Tess of the D'Urbervilles and spend my days mashing up turnips to make ends meet. Under my fetching peasant smock, my tummy would bulge ignominiously and I'd finally grow too tired to mash the turnips and I'd sink into penury. The goth would be told – I didn't even know his surname – and he would be banished to the

Colonies to flee the shame, his sugared hair becoming sadly limp and flat in the tropical heat. Hard to believe that a teenager in the 1980s could be lying in bed having these thoughts, but hey, that's Catholicism for you.

I felt sick for two days, another sure-fire confirmation of my condition, and the only person I confided in was Lucy. She was really supportive and promised that she would come away and live with me in the countryside. She felt responsible somehow – it was her sofa that my baby had been conceived on after all. She was also quite keen to know the details of what had actually happened.

'I can't remember anything except for the smell of smoky bacon.'

A pause. Lucy nodded thoughtfully. 'Yeah, apparently it does.'

Lucy said that she would earn enough money for the two of us and the baby – she was keen to set up a jewellery and bead shop, and luckily, had already started collecting feathers and little glass balls.

Lucy and I bought the pregnancy kit together and it was with a sick heart and hunched shoulders that I sat in Lucy's parents' bathroom with it there in front of me. Doing it in my house would have been madness – Mum, with her wolverine sixth-sense, would have sniffed out in a trice that there was foul play occurring in her lavatory. When no blue line appeared in the little hatch, I cried tears of relief and Lucy and I jumped up and down hugging each other. Our lives were free again! We could stay in the city! I think secretly Lucy was quite disappointed that her jewellery business wasn't going to get the kick-start it needed, but she soon cheered up. I promised her there and then that I would never ever end up being compromised by a) drink or b) a diddy-goth again. Ever. We toasted that with two Purple Parachutes.

As I sat in the loo in Dr Sweeting's surgery, I realised that of course I was pregnant. My period was late, I'd been smelling phantom asparagus for days, been on all fours by a dual carriageway and cried at a clown. When the tester-kit was cooked and I saw the thin blue line in the hatch all that kept going through my mind was, 'Of course I am. I could have told you that!'

Poor Dr Sweeting's little suit got a real dousing, as I cried on to her shoulder-pads like a big baby. She gave me a whole load of leaflets and

I practically ran all the way home I was so excited and over-emotional. Then I suddenly stopped running. I was terrified that the baby was going to fall out.

226 days to go ...

WE'VE BEEN IN A HAZE for most of today. Dan went the colour of the Rigoletto when I told him the epic news last night. He fell back into his chair and was pretty speechless for a couple of minutes. He looked at the pregnancy lolly-stick with the blue line in the hatch as bold as the day and he couldn't quite believe it.

'And you're sure the blue line means you're pregnant?'

'Yes, isn't urine amazing?'

'You're sure it hasn't been left too long and it's measured your cholesterol level by mistake?'

'No!'

'So we're probably going to have a baby in about eight months?'

'Yes.'

'Our baby will be with us in this flat in thirty-two weeks?'

'If all goes well, yes.'

'And you're sure it's your pregnancy test – it didn't get mixed up with anybody else's?'

'Dan, are you OK?'

'I'm absolutely fine. I'm ... I'm ...'

His bottom lip starts to wobble, then he coughs loudly. Then he slaps his thighs. His voice veers up and down like a pubescent choirboy: 'I've always wanted to be called Daddy.'

225 days to go ...

I STILL FEEL SICK and sleepy but it doesn't matter today. I feel like I've been gently guided in a waltz by large invisible hands for most of the day, gliding around the place as if I were on castors. I can't concentrate on anything much, I graze on what I find in the fridge, try to focus on work, think about phoning people up to tell them our news but decide not to and then spend a lot of time in front of the mirror analysing my bust. And all the while I keep brimming with tears at the thought of this lifeform taking root inside of me.

Dan phones in from work. 'Are you all right? Are you getting enough rest?'

'I think so. The most energetic thing I've done today is unwrap a Penguin biscuit.'

'Look, I've been on the Internet. Don't eat any prawns, soft cheese or pâté. Or peanuts!'

And then twenty minutes later. 'It's me.'

'Good. Me here too.'

'Just been on the net again. If you're going to have a bath, don't make it too hot. It can be dangerous, especially if you've just drunk gin.'

'I'll keep that in mind.'

'And oh, probably best not drink any gin whatever. Hey, sorry if I'm being bossy.'

'No, you're not being bossy. Just insistent.'

'I'm so proud of you.'

'And me of you. See you this evening.'

It feels as though I'm barely off the phone when it rings again.

'Sweetheart, it's me. Dan. Look I may be barking up the wrong tree here, but I've been on the net again. I've found something quite interesting. It says that babies respond to Mozart really well in the womb. Something to do with the rhythm. Maybe you could listen to Mozart's *Requiem* today? We've got it on CD upstairs. Just a thought.'

'Dan, my love, you are now being a little bossy and I'm not sure if its ears are big enough to hear yet, anyway. It's only about a centimetre long, if that.'

'You're absolutely right, sorry to disturb.'

Then it can't be more than fifteen minutes later.

'Ginger!'

'No, it's Mel.'

'Ginger! Ginger for sickness! I've been out and I've got a whole load of it. It's really good for nausea! Byee!'

Five minutes later the phone rings. Gordon Bennett. I pick it up and shout, 'Don't tell me, you're bringing me charcoal for my wind!'

'Mel?'

It's my mother.

'What's this about wind? Are you all right, darling? You're not expecting, are you?'

Just hearing my mum at the other end of the line can reduce me to quivering sobs on an average day. But now that I've got a wave of hormones the size of the Norfolk Wash coursing through my system it's Game Over as soon as I hear a whiff of her voice. And how on earth does she possess that voodoo intuition thing? It's ludicrous how she manages to work out what's going on. In between sobs, I tell her that yes, I am to be a mother and then literally howl down the line. When I've calmed down and she's assimilated the news and reported it to Dad, we get down to the nitty-gritty.

'I'll send you some literature that'll help, darling.'

'Not the book about contraception written by that bishop?' (It had always sat on the top shelf in the bathroom.)

'No, darling, I think it's too late for contraception, don't you? I'll send you some sound practical mothering stuff.'

I suspect she's referring to her Bible – *The Mothercraft Manual*. And manual is the right word; it's like a car maintenance handbook. It might have been the acme of good advice in the 1950s, but I'm dearly hoping that things have moved on since then.

'Congratulations, my darling, lots of love to you both.'

And then, I'm afraid the howling starts up again. Even more than before. Once I've collected myself I manage to say, 'M … M … Mum, thank you for being s … s … such a g … g … good m … m …'

There is silence. 'Mum?'

Nothing.

'Mum!'

I am met with an empty phone-line. Full respect to the woman. She hung up on her baying wreck of a daughter. I hope I'd do the same.

224 days to go ...

It's funny how the most momentous life-changing events can be forever linked with absolute trivia. I will always associate getting pregnant for the first time with Dr Sweeting's fragrant shoulder-pads. A builder that did our damp-proofing was a massive Elvis fan and once said to me as the kettle boiled, 'The day the King went was a tragedy. I was washing my dog at the time. Didn't rinse out the soap properly. Gave him a very matted appearance.'

My uncle was in Dallas the day that JFK was shot, but the thing he remembers most about that shocking day was the hors d'oeuvres in his hotel: 'Watercress soup we were served. In the middle of Texas, extraordinary!'

It must be nature's shock absorber. The enormity of what is going to happen to us in eight months' time is just too much to take on board, but thankfully the power of detail (and the shoulder-pad) has obscured everything.

'Do you think we'll need to widen the doors?' I ask out of nowhere.

We're both lounging in the living room, silently caught in our own reflections on the future.

'What?'

'They just look really narrow.'

Dan whips out his tape measure, which he has rather sinisterly taken to keeping attached to his belt, along with his mobile phone.

'Hmm. Thirty inches across. D'you reckon you'll be wider than that?'

'Dunno, could be as big as a house.'

'Mel, you're not saying we should move house?'

220 days to go ...

THANK GOD, the morning sickness seems to have receded a little, or perhaps I've just become accustomed to it. I don't know where the 'morning' bit comes from though. Mine's an all-day bonanza. It's like having a permanent light car-sickness – a kind of salivary feeling in my mouth, as if I'm in a new saloon car, with that smell of plastic, being driven a little too fast and smoothly. Actually, just thinking about it is making me feel sick so I'd better stop. I can deal with it as long as I keep a dry cracker to hand. And as long as I don't look at that bloody car parked outside. Even if I see just a snatch of it out of the corner of my eye – its silhouette out there on the roadside, its silly cream interior – I want to heave. Even the word 'Rigoletto' is making me feel queasy. We're going to have to sell it – I have to talk to Dan the minute he's back.

What am I saying? Of *course* we'll have to sell it. It's a two-seater twat-mobile – where the hell's the nipper going to sit?

Welcome to parenthood. Stage one: lose your stylish, impractical jalopy and purchase a nice, supermarket-friendly hatchback with mechanised wing-mirrors and a back windscreen that de-mists properly. This I accept, but hear me now, I will *never* display a Baby on Board sticker in the back of my car. Or one of those ridiculous animal shades that you stick on the side window. Never. And I will never have a back window full of toys or a silly fake steering-wheel attached to the back of the driver's seat so that Baby can drive along too. Good. I feel better for getting that off my chest. Speaking of which, they are definitely bigger.

219 days to go ...

'DO YOU THINK they're bigger, Dan?'

This is about the fortieth time I've asked him this question this morning. I'd noticed as I dressed that my knockers were slightly straining out of their cups and creating that lovely bisected four-bosomed look through my jumper.

'I mean, look at them from this angle.' I jut the rack upwards like a prim 1950s underwear model.

'Look, Mel, I'm a bloke and if I do that with my flat chest it looks like *I've* got tits.' Poor Dan is exasperated but does the action anyway just to demonstrate. He's right – it does sort of give him breasts.

'No, but look! Even if I hunch over like this, they're still bigger.' I adopt the Quasimodo position. 'Maybe not exactly bigger as in bigger cup size, but just kind of bigger heavier. They're heavier, that's what it is. Do you think I've put on weight, Dan?'

He's now deep into the sports section of his newspaper but even his devotion to the England cricket team cannot have blocked out my question.

'It depends on what you mean by weight,' comes the answer from behind the paper.

'Well, I suppose I mean, do you, in any way, shape or form, think that I am in any way heavier, porkier, chubbier? Have I stacked it on? Come on, be honest.'

'Maybe a bit.'

'But I'm only a few weeks pregnant, Dan! I've been eating exactly the same so far!'

'You said be honest. You *could* be carrying more weight.'

'And does "carrying weight" mean that I've put it on? Do I *look* fatter, Dan? Or do I just look tired because I'm laden down? Tired or fat?'

'A bit, yes.'

'Which one? Tired?'

'No, a bit … you know, the other thing you said.'

'WHAT? But I've been eating exactly the same. It's winter too and people always look fatter in winter. It's the light and the colours and layers we all wear. I'm also probably not moving around as much and I'm definitely retaining water. I feel full of water. But I don't think I look fatter. My clothes are a bit tighter but I don't think I am, per se, bigger. Am I?'

'Hmm?'

'Dan?'

Dan sighs. He and the sports section have become crumpled and dejected.

'No. No. No, you're not.'

'Now you're lying! Dan, come on, be honest and tell me that I haven't put on weight.'

'No, you haven't put on weight.'

He snaps the paper back up in front of his face. I look into the mirror and smooth myself.

'I knew I hadn't.'

218 days to go ...

PAWEL, OUR ELUSIVE LODGER, returned from Poland today. He's been back home for a couple of months, and I really must say that Dan and I have loved having the place to ourselves. Though he's a lovely bloke, Pawel – PhD student, very quiet, rather intense, very low maintenance.

He did his usual thing, which was to creep very carefully into the flat at about five in the morning, having got on the coach in Warsaw twenty hours previously. He always places some carefully wrapped waxy packages in the fridge, containing very salty cheese and garlicky sausage. And he always puts a bottle of Zubrowka vodka for us in the freezer compartment. Normally I'd be blissfully unaware of all this until I saw his face coyly smiling though his moustache around the kitchen door at breakfast time. Not today. My new-found, extra-sensory, bat-like ears picked up the brush of his softly soled academic's shoe the minute it sponged up the pathway towards the front door. I heard his magician-like insertion and deft turning of the key in the lock, and his panther-like movement through the flat to his room. One of my eyes had flicked fully open as soon as I heard him and my eyebrow arched like a church window as I sensed ... yes, *sensed* his presence. My nostril sniffed delicately above the duvet. I could tell where he was in his room, exactly what he was doing and what he was planning to do. I could have run down the corridor, jumped into his room in full growl and pinned him against his wardrobe with an enormous lioness paw. This was cool. I was queen of the jungle lying on my rock. When I couldn't get back to sleep, however, the lioness in me disappeared and the fishwife reared her head again.

I saw Pawel at seven for a cup of tea and I'm afraid I was pretty grouchy. He's not a big conversationalist at the best of times and when I'm with him I end up carrying out a sort of two-way chat all by myself. Dan says it's nerves and I should just be happy with some silence between us, but I hate silence. It makes me feel nervous. It's like dead air-space on a radio show. One second of it can feel like a minute.

'Hi there, Pawel, welcome back to London.'

'Good morning.'

'Did you have a good time in Warsaw? Did you get all your stuff done?'

'I think yes.'

'Great. And was the journey OK? I should imagine it was quite trafficky, wasn't it, and were your family all right? You were seeing quite a few of them, weren't you? Yes, there's quite a lot of you, from all over the country, meeting up, I think you were.'

'Yes.'

'And all's fine here, Pawel! Yes, work's going well, we've been a bit lazy, you know, haven't got very much done in the last couple of weeks.'

A pause.

'But I'm starting a new presenting job. Should be quite fun. And Dan's got his translating. So it's all go. Milk with the tea? No, you always have lemon. So you'll be getting back to your studies, I suppose. Going well, is it? You work so hard I'm sure it is.'

A longish pause, which is more than I can bear, and then he says, 'Goodbye', gives a slight bow – and that's the last we'll see of him for the rest of the day. He always comes in after nine at night and studies till well into the small hours.

I specifically fail to mention our real news. I come over all girly. I can't face it. It's just too personal for our strange relationship. I'm sure the feeling's mutual. I imagine he'd just bow and leave the room. It sometimes feels as though we live in a nineteenth-century country house.

Pawel is like a friendly unseen spectre in the flat, but we're going to have to tell him the news so that he can find a new place to live because we'll need the space for the baby's room. Wow. That is one hell of a weird concept. Pawel is soon to be replaced by a little froggy person in a towelling sleeping suit. I suddenly have in my mind's eye a dear little baby but with Pawel's sphinx-like expression, moustache and slightly greasy fine hair plastered down on its forehead. Time for a kip I think.

217 days to go ...

I'M HAVING TO KEEP the crackers going at a fairly constant rate at the moment. I feel like my granny. She always used to eat dry crackers and her voice would click when she talked. As soon as my mouth's empty it fills with that car-sick salivary feeling. Not pleasant. I haven't actually thrown up recently but boy, do I feel like I'm about to. There is a pile of Pawel's washing which is making me feel really green around the gills. He's meticulously clean but there's a shirt in there, the one he travelled in, that smells deep-fried. I can barely go near it. I hoik it up on the end of a broom-handle and flick it towards the washing machine.

The Mothercraft Manual arrives in the post today, and Mum's written a little note:

> Darling!
>
> I hear they're recommending Mozart for babies in the womb. I wouldn't take it any further dear. Certainly no Wagner or Beethoven at this crucial stage of your confinement. We don't want Baby to develop German tendencies do we? What do the experts say about a little Vaughan Williams, or Elgar? Surely they can only be good for Baby?
>
> All love
> Mum xxxx

Once I free *The Mothercraft Manual* from its over-zealous packing, I see a smiling lady with one gloved hand resting protectively over her stomach while the other strokes the bars of a cot. She's wearing a head-scarf, yes, and the ends are tied jauntily under one ear. Her cheeks are as red as little apples and even though there is an obvious bump emerging under her large A-line smock top, she's still wearing very high stiletto heels.

Along with the usual bills, the postman also handed me a manila envelope that contained the contract for *Ex Maniac*. I'm torn. I don't know if I should sign it. Do I want this? But the chance to flesh out the old bank account before the baby arrives is too good to refuse. I sign on the various dotted lines and decide to get on with phoning my closest friends. It's about time I shared our news with someone.

216 days to go ...

I SPENT ABOUT FIVE HOURS on the phone yesterday. Not because we've got hundreds and hundreds of close friends, but because I wanted to speak to the ones who really count for hours and hours. On reflection I might have become a bit of a bore. I did that thing where you make a little gag and then you repeat the same gag in the story every time you tell it – 'Pregnant? I thought I just had a terrible case of PMT!' Now it's not very funny I'll admit, but it went down quite well with the first person so I kept the little routine going. By the eleventh call, 'Pregnant? I thought I just had a terrible case of PMT!' was pretty polished and I'd even added a semi-improvised little laugh between the two phrases. I talked at an old college friend for thirty-five minutes, then phoned straight back because I'd left something out – to do with lateness of periods or something – and I got his answering machine straight away. The penny dropped. People care, but nobody cares *that* much. Then I rang Mum, as a tester.

'Hi, Mum, it's me!'

'Hello, darling. Now, how are you? How are you feeling?'

'I'm OK, pretty euphoric still. I'm not sleeping though.'

'Now, Melly, I know what you're like with your sleep. You must get lots and lots of rest or you'll be useless.'

'You're so right, Mum. I feel half asleep, I suppose. A sort of semi-sleep where I sense everything that's going on in the house.'

'Mmmm.'

'I feel great though. I still can't quite believe it. I've started to tell close mates – everyone's so delighted.'

'That's nice.'

'I'm not going to tell everyone. It's just so hard to keep it to myself.'

'Mmmm.'

I get the message loud and clear.

The horror. I'm already a fully functioning mother-to-be bore.

215 days to go ...

GOOD NEWS. The Rigoletto has gone. Dan sold it to a friend of a friend who came to collect it wearing a beret and blouson leather jacket. A perfect match.

The bad news is that Dan has replaced it with a hatchback. A Nissan-bloody-Micra to be exact. Mode of transport-elect to the terminally safety conscious. Oh God. I suddenly have a vision of myself in fifteen years' time, waiting in this very same car in the middle of the night. I'll be in full tweeds, parked up and listening to Radio 3 outside some terrible teenage party where inside my kids are getting up to God knows what – throwing up into an airing cupboard? Nude fumbling in a spare room? Oh the arguments, lies, tantrums and denials that are going to fill this boring old hatchback.

214 days to go ...

SO HOW FAR GONE AM I? It's an awful expression – 'far gone' – sounds like I've lost my mind, which I can assure you is still very much intact. A bit spongy maybe. How long have I been in the club for? How far up the stick am I? How cooked is the bun in my oven? Blimey, they're all awful. The worst has got to be 'in the family way'. What a pointless British beating around of the bush. It's like asking someone who's dying if they're 'in the funeral way'. Come on, let's call a spade a ruddy spade. I'm pregnant. Actually, I don't much care for that word either because of a girl at primary school called Nancy who used to bully me. Preg-Nancy. It reminds me of having my shins kicked. Perhaps I shall have to resort to using the phrase used in *The Mothercraft Manual* – 'expecting'. I bet the Royal Family say 'expecting', however. I may look like one of the Windsors after a rough night on the sauce, but I'm not sure I want to sound like one of them.

213 days to go ...

'DAN?'

Every time I say this I notice poor Dan wince ever so slightly, as if he knows he's about to enter the mine-filled territory that is How To Answer Your Pregnant Partner Without Upsetting Her. But he must also beware that his answers stay the right side of molly-coddling, fuss-budgeting or just plain patronising.

'Yes?' he replies, every atom of his being bristling and wondering what's coming next.

'When do you think the baby was actually conceived?'

Phew. Relief is visible in his face. No questions about weight. Or: Has my face got older? Do I look more serious? Have I lost my sense of humour? Do I look greyer? Do you think I'm beginning to look more like my mother?

'Hmmm. The conception. Well, when were we last really drunk?'

My face falls. What a sad testament to our sex-life.

'No! Mel! By that I didn't mean that we have to get really wasted before we have sex – you know that I still love you when I'm sober. But, well, you know what I mean. This was an accident.'

'An accident? Dan, that sounds so negative!' I say, a serious frown setting in.

'You're right,' he checks quickly, 'accident's totally the wrong word. I mean surprise. Happy surprise!'

It really was a surprise to both of us, like every working couple in their thirties these days who are living that kind of settled, rather smug existence of being in control of their little world – anally planning everything to the nth degree. (What are we doing six weekends from now? Hang on, I'll just have to check the diary ... No, sorry, we can't make the WOMAD Festival that weekend – we're going to Barcelona!)

I blush when I think of how we used to discuss becoming parents. We'd decided to start thinking about planning to start thinking about having a baby in the window between the Edinburgh Festival and the start of Dan's trip to the Krakow Film Festival in October. How smug is it to plan your baby between two arts festivals? Not to mention the arrogance of just assuming that our baby will be fertilised, willy-nilly, on the exact day that we prescribe! We've become too used to having our life on a gastro-plate.

These days most people like to plan their first baby to coincide with a degree of financial stability, which seems reasonable to me. But I have to say that I did almost punch a guy at an awful party once when he announced that he'd have to be making sixty grand a year before he even considered starting a family. His poor wife was standing next to him as he said it, the hope in her eyes turning to ashes. I felt so sorry for her – it was unbelievably crass of him to put a price on her dreams of having a baby. I often think of the two of them and wonder if she's managed to engineer a little 'accident' somehow. Not by pricking little holes into the condom, no, just pricking holes into him and then finding someone decent to have a baby with.

Mixing babies and money talk is a mug's game. Dan and I sat down last night and did a bit of accounting. We worked out that we need to be on Elton John-type salaries to pay for this child for the next thirty years. Even the basics – baby gear, food, trainers, toys, holidays, childcare, university tuition fees, driving lessons, paying for their wedding, possible prison bail, help with first house and all food consumed over the next three decades – makes for a terrifying prospect. And I'm sure there are plenty of hidden extras we haven't even accounted for. What about Christmas? We decided after much hysterical and rather nervous laughter that the only way of tackling it is day by day. Look at it as a hire purchase agreement rather than the full payment up front. If not, you might as well be wheeled direct from the maternity unit to the psychiatric ward.

I love hearing the tales of my parents' generation. They were so much more romantic, so much more laissez-faire about the whole thing. My mum and dad didn't save up for years before they got married – they just did it because they loved each other. My dad borrowed fifty quid to buy a car so that he could take my mum on their honeymoon to Cornwall. How dashing is that? OK, so the car broke down just outside London and they spent the next two weeks in Mousehole rowing, but isn't the idea of it lovely?

Artist friends of my mum's didn't have a bean to rub between them when they had their first baby. For the first few months of his life the little lad slept in a chest of drawers. This might sound la-di-da and just too fey for words, but I do think it shows up my generation to be just a bunch of over-cautious, scaredy-cat hedge-betters. At least that's my feeling right now. My new state has today filled me with new punch and feist. But who knows what retreat tomorrow will bring?

212 days to go ...

WE HAVE FINALLY WORKED out when the baby must have been conceived, and Dan's right, it does happen to coincide with rather a lot of alcohol. An old schoolfriend of mine got married and Dan and I took the opportunity to get completely hoovered at her reception. So much so that Dan actually thought he was managing to converse with the groom's father in his native Armenian tongue. What he was actually doing – and I remember because I knocked over a massive tray of quiche I was laughing so much – was speaking in English but very loudly and with a very slurred made-for-TV Russian accent. We left the wedding reception late and staggered towards the nearest bank where I tried to get money out of the cashpoint machine with my shoe. When we got home, let's just say that the 'contra' was very much left out of the 'ception' equation.

Forgive me for sounding twee around the subject of sex. My Catholic upbringing means that I still think Jilly Cooper is a 'racy' writer for goodness' sake, and the closest I've ever come to watching a porn film was *Carry On Emmanuelle.*

After my crucial trip to the loo, Dr Sweeting had stemmed my tears by getting out a special wheel. Actually it was more like a wheel within a wheel and she used it rather mysteriously to work out when the conception was likely to have fallen, working from the date of my last period. It's all very complicated and I'm starting to envy Kate and her yellow-penned diary 'O' days. Dan and I finally managed to fudge it together. I am somewhere around the eight-week mark. We think. Two months gone already. That's nearly a quarter of the way through! We must tell Pawel that he's going to have to leave. We must plan the baby's room. I must swot up on the childbirth literature. I must buy some bigger bras. I must embrace the hatchback car. We must change the house. I must learn to knit and sew and create potato print paintings. I must learn how to bath a baby. And feed it. And look after it. OH MY GOD!

211 days to go ...

I WAS ON THE RADIO TODAY. Pretty basic fayre – contributing to a live show called *Women on the Waves.* Not a history of female seafarers – although I could have provided the right outfit for the occasion – but the story of women on radio. The really exciting thing, though, was that a certain National Treasure, someone I've always been dying to meet, was a fellow guest. She was already at the studio when I arrived, resplendent in a symphony of salmon and avocado including pashmina and showbusiness slacks. I found it hard not to throw myself at her feet and kiss her cameo brooch, but managed to keep my professionalism intact. We went On Air but I felt more like a member of the audience as I listened in awe to her anecdotes. But all was not well.

I had been filled all morning with the most insufferable, bilious, grey feeling of nausea. It had started in the minicab on the way into the station. The driver had one of those Smelly Tree things hanging over the dashboard and I had to stick my head out of the back window like a big old hound to avoid its sweet-smelling horridness. My mouth was slippery with saliva, my teeth felt spongy and I had an overwhelming desire to ... I just shut my eyes and mouthed a mantra over and over to myself: 'Cleansing Mints. Cutting through! Cleansing Mints. Cutting through!' I just had to keep imagining a rush of liquid mint coursing through my mouth, with myself surfing its crest. It had gradually subsided, but as soon as I was in the stuffy studio, the feeling returned – lurking like a mugger in the shadows.

The radio host asked the National Treasure a fittingly reverential question.

'So when did you first realise that you could make people ... make people ...'

With a suddenness that shocked me, the acrid wave rose from the pit of my stomach. An arc of hot vomit leapt from my mouth and splattered the microphone. My first chunder live on air.

The National Treasure wasn't remotely phased. She had just sat there and watched proceedings with genteel interest.

'What's that, dear? When was the first time I made someone throw up? Ooh, it was probably during the war. I had a terrible routine with some other dancers. We called ourselves the Little Pickles and we were dreadful.'

Her sheer professionalism took my breath away, what was left of it.

210 days to go ...

I'M TRYING TO COME to terms with these oral explosions. I spoke to my sister Kate on the phone and she told me that her sickness only lasted four months. *Only* four months! Blimey, that seems like an eternity. As Tony Hancock might have said if he had ever been pregnant – that's got to be at least two hundred pints of sick.

Kate's going to leave her kids with us for a night when she and her partner Jake go off for his parents' wedding anniversary do. I feel guilty. I love my niece and nephew to distraction but I've barely given them a moment's thought these last few weeks. It's been all me, me, me.

209 days to go ...

DAN IS DOING a lot of measuring at the moment. It's his way of getting mentally prepared.

We went to the pub last night and I made my poor husband take me home at 9 p.m. I just started yawning and the table had that sharp vinegary whiff like it had been wiped with a rank cloth. I keep sniffing at everything around me like a police dog, which is a bit unnerving. I even started sniffing at the bar and the barman looked embarrassed and checked his armpits. This is going to be a nightmare.

208 days to go ...

TODAY WE BOTH WENT DOWN TO our local bookshop to get a book on how to give birth. Of course, I know the basic principles – large baby must somehow emerge from comparatively small hole – but we both feel in need of some cold facts and warm reassurances from wise but friendly best-selling experts. I know some of these mandatory tomes because parents to be tend to leave them ostentatiously and casually out alongside their week-end *Guardian* or the latest Booker Prize nominee. It really is only the basics I know. I spent most of the time in O-level Biology trying to burn Mary Flynn's lab coat or showing off, like a good little entertainer, while the man's genitals were displayed on an overhead slide-projector.

Buying the literature is all well and good, but with my current concentration levels, reading it will be another matter. I've got the focus of a gnat. And it's got decidedly worse in the last few days: I can't even read the captions underneath the photos in *Hello!* magazine. I just flick, flit, flick over the photos like one of those hovering insects that lurk around ditches. Apparently once you have the baby, the longest thing you'll probably read is a Ladybird book anyway.

Dan, in his own male way, is particularly keen on getting the litera-ture in. Like his beloved car manuals, he sees it as a way of bringing order to the chaos, light to our angst-filled darkness.

There are so many books to choose from and every angle is covered – feeding baby organically, same-sex parenting, weaving for baby, how to get the genius out of your child, how to get the poo out of your child, singing to your foetus, how to love labour, the loving birth, the loving family. And one book for fathers. I'm beginning to learn that fathers tend to get a rough deal. In the NHS pamphlet Dr Sweeting gave me there is one page entitled 'Making Dad Feel Involved' in which they simply tell you to give him the odd hug. Simple.

I head over to 'Dad' to see how he's getting on, having decided on a sensible book written by a sensible ex-TV doctor, with loads of diagrams, a glossary of terms and a Q & A section. Hopefully it can answer the really vital issues like 'How do I get rid of my back breasts?' and 'What to do if your baby looks like Paul Daniels'. Dan has been totally immersed, thumbing through book after book, and lingering rather too long over a breast-feeding manual. When I nudge him, he's studiously assessing *Baby Lives with Jenny and Sarah.*

'Look! There's a close-up of the baby's head coming out! ... and there's a great recipe for flapjacks too.'

207 days to go ...

TODAY I GRABBED a whole wodge of mother and baby-type mags at WH Smith – probably more suited to my attention span. And typically, while the sensible lady doctor's spin remains unspun this morning, I can't get enough of a special pull-out feature in one of my glossies – the Perfect Popstar Pregnancy or as the banner line has it: 'From Number Ones to Number Twos!' The article is awash with star tips, advice, cautionary tales, regimes and where to buy a Louis Vuitton leather papoose. It's jammed full of shots of stars in crop tops and trainers with their perfect peachy and glistening bulges sticking out over combat trousers. They look stunning. This is how you want to look when you're pregnant – fecund not fat. Glowing, trendy and full-to-bursting with that special type of all-natural, mother-to-be hormone energy. It's ridiculous, but I'm smitten. I want to be a yummy celebrity mummy. Or as Dan rather too keenly described them, and their showy, skinny look, Bare Mini-mums.

The thing about being a Bare Mini-mum is that you actually have to be both mini and bare before you get pregnant. As a healthily sized female I am neither mini nor will I bare anything except ankles and wrists unless there's quite a lot of darkness and/or alcohol involved. How I even began to suppose that I could in any way equate my pregnancy experience with a popstar's baffles me. Most of these women are in their mid-twenties and have gravity on their side. I am thirty-three and gravity is not only on my side but on my thighs, my knees, my chin, my jowls and my upper arms.

Nevertheless, I dig out a pair of Dan's old combat trousers. I then chop up a T-shirt to make it into a croptop, put on a pair of sporty little plimsolls and crown the whole thing off with what I thought was a pair of gamine little pigtails. I'm afraid one look in the mirror confirms my suspicions – Care in the Community. Or a marine who has gone to a fancy dress party as a Spice Girl. We don't possess a full-length mirror, so I am balancing precariously on a chair in front of the hall mirror when who should come through the front door but Pawel.

These moments should be private.

'Oh hi, Pawel, I'm just dusting ... and ... I've been trying out a new look. How have you been? We haven't seen much of you recently! We must have a chat sometime, catch up. Look at me up on this chair! Quite dangerous really.'

Pawel mumbles 'Good evening' through his moustache, bows and shuffles up to his room.

206 days to go ...

THERE'S A MESSAGE on the answering machine from Amanda. She must have picked up my call at last. What we mere minions refer to as August is for Amanda 'Majorca month'. Or is it Malta? I can never remember. She must be about eight months pregnant by now and I really felt I should get in touch. I've been 'friends' with Amanda since we were three. Our mums knew each other from church and the Leatherhead coffee-morning circuit. Amanda and I sang in the choir and did our First Holy Communion together. She upstaged all us girls at that particular event when she wore a white satin hooped dress with matching handbag, veil and head-dress. And the prime object of my envy – white patent shoes! I begged for an outfit like Amanda's but Mum said that God wasn't interested in our outfits, only in our souls.

'But Amanda's got shiny soles!' I wailed. Mum hrrmphed and put me in a white smock and T-bar sandals.

Amanda's family lived at the posh end of Leatherhead, where the houses had stone lions on plinths at their gates. Her dad owned the local chain of laundrettes and the taxi firm. They were loaded, so Amanda was sent to the local private girls' school, Parsonage Mead, which the rest of us called 'Parsnips Weed'.

Still, I loved going round to Amanda's house. We were allowed fizzy drinks from their Soda Stream. She had birthday parties in their indoor swimming pool, and her Dad got her a real pony for her eleventh birthday. That was before he 'disappeared' for a few months. Amanda told me he'd gone to Spain to set up more laundrettes, but Mum said he was inside and that we had to pray for him.

As teenagers we played Eurovision Song Contest and she always got to play the really glamorous countries like France or Luxembourg. I was inevitably Turkey and she always made sure that I lost. It was a very unfair system actually – there was no jury. We simply argued it out between the two of us.

'Look Mel, I'm a much better singer than you and my French entry is so much better than your Turkish one.'

'How do you know? You don't understand Turkish, Mandy!'

'Well you don't understand it either, Mel. What does "Hom Buddy Ominum" actually mean? Doesn't sound very Turkish to me.'

'But it's not fair, Mandy. France always wins!'

'Because France is best and my song was best!'

At which point she proceeded to drown me out by singing her winning French entry, which went something like 'Oh May Mi May Moi!' and then performed some really twee dance moves to go with it.

And that's how our relationship has stayed, pretty much. Amanda still considers herself a winner and I just tag along with what she wants when I happen to get roped into her games. She runs a very successful chain of gyms, and is personal trainer to the odd famous person too.

'I was out jogging with Robbie the other day,' she'll drop casually into the conversation.

'Oh yes?' you reply, trying to sound as cool as possible about her pop-starry connections.

'Robbie's such a great guy and he's lost tons of weight.'

She's holding that celebrity carrot out so tantalisingly that you simply have to ask.

'Robbie Williams! What's he like?'

'No! Rob Curling! Used to be on Newsroom South East. Used to go out with thingy-bob that used to be in EastEnders.'

Amanda loves celebrity. She's obsessed with all the celeb mags and the best day of her life was when she was photographed by a paparazzi while doing burpees in the park with Matthew Kelly. She has it lavishly framed and hanging in her hall.

Dan thinks she's hilarious and we never turn down an invite to a dinner party at Amanda's, thankfully a once-in-a-blue-moon occurrence because we really do have very little in common. I quietly detest her friends and scorn her lifestyle. While she vocally pities mine. I suppose I put up with her out of duty to our past. The last time we went round for dinner was a classic.

'Hi Mandy!' I greet her.

'It's Manda,' she says through smiling gritted teeth.

'You'll always be good old Mandy from Leatherhead to me!' I protest, so that everyone inside can hear.

'You lived in Leatherhead,' she snaps, 'we lived on the Esher borders.'

And with that she ushers me firmly into her Moroccan-inspired living room. Amanda's whole house looks as if one too many TV makeover shows have been let loose on it. Each room with a distinct theme groans under the weight of over-styling – the Provençal Country Kitchen awash with gingham and stencilling, the Minimalist Dining area with its uncompromising chrome table and chairs, the Middle Eastern yoga room full of heavy brass lanterns and swirling batique – even the loo's hilariously called Bognor, and is cluttered with English seaside ornaments: buckets, shells and cheeky postcards.

Amanda feels safe with themes. Dinner tonight has a sort of Tuscan theme with a burnt orange look to the fore. We all start with grappa cocktails. 'Sting drinks this on his Tuscan estate!' Amanda informs us intimately, like she's ever met him. Amanda places orange Tuscan bean hotpot in orange bowls onto orange plates on orange raffia table-mats. There are floating orange candles everywhere, and orange petals have been thrown casually over everyone's seats.

Her husband Roger is marked by his absence as usual. I think I've only ever clapped eyes on him once in my life. He owns several tennis clubs and is always abroad on business.

We make a motley party, masticating on our beans round Mandy's chrome table. There's a hairdresser called James with a ridiculous mane of dyed auburn hair, a stick-thin PR woman called Tash, several very buff fitness instructors who grin all evening and a businesswoman called Emma who takes five mobile-phone calls through dinner. Everyone is tanned and clinks with bling the size of loo chains.

'God I think Posh's new hair extensions are fab!' says James.

'I think they're tacky,' proffers Tash.

'Well get me the details for the meeting tomorrow!' shouts Emma into her mobile.

'I've met Posh's personal trainer,' gloats Amanda, 'and apparently David doesn't like them either so Posh has agreed to have them cut off.'

'Ooooh!' says James, rubbing his podgy hands, and so it continues while Dan and I get quietly drunk.

By the time coffee arrives we've adjourned to Amanda's Seventies-themed snug – all white furry rugs, onyx ashtrays and a fake fire. The conversation turns to Prince Andrew.

'I think he's fab,' says James.

'Oh no!' says Tash. 'He's so chunky!'

'He's actually lost loads of weight,' says Amanda confidentially, 'he's off the carbs apparently,' and everyone nods their heads reverently.

These people are starting to make me feel slightly itchy and I suddenly feel a terrible desire to throw red wine all over Amanda's white suede sofa. Then all eyes turn to me as James says, 'So tell us, Mel, you must have met a fair few minor celebs in your time. You used to be one yourself!'

The red wine has rendered me tongue-fuddled. I want to reply with something Dorothy Parker would have been proud of, but all I can come up with is a useless ruddy-faced grin.

Inside I'm stung. 'Used to'! The big-haired buffoon hasn't even given me the accolade of the present tense!

I'm pretty drunk by the time we leave and I get my own back on James by directing the international sign for 'tosser' at him as we leave. I do it in the hall at an angle so that nobody can see me but him. He puts his frilly cuff up to his mouth in genuine horror.

I am adamant in the taxi on the way home that we're never going to Amanda's for dinner ever again. Dan says we've been saying that for fifteen years.

Even though she bugs the living daylights out of me, I suppose life wouldn't be quite the same without Amanda's occasional presence. I get up to find her number.

200 days to go ...

NOT MUCH NAUSEA TODAY, which is a blessed relief. But it has been replaced by an ominous new sensation: an aching, yawning chasm of emptiness. Now there is nothing wrong with this if you really feel like you've deserved this hunger – after, say, a 20-mile hike in the depths of winter. If, however, you have done nothing all morning except sit at your computer supposedly working, but in reality playing some pretty fierce rounds of Snake, then this feeling is a bit of a worry.

I see off a dozen slices of buttery toast, then the remains of the weekend's quiche beckons me from the fridge, before I finally settle back at my computer with a fresh packet of Club biscuits and a 2-litre bottle of Coke. It's only ten o'clock. In the morning.

But I'm pregnant! For once in my life I have the perfect excuse! I'm perfectly entitled to eat that snack, in fact I *must* because there is a hungry little mouth in there who must be fed too and if you don't eat that snack, he or she will probably fade away.

At least, that's what I had thought until I consulted the – rapidly becoming the bane of my life – sensible TV lady doctor. I could hardly believe what I was reading: 'You should add 500 calories to your normal daily intake.' That's pathetic! That's only seven custard creams! That's not eating for one, never mind two.

Foodwise, there are two categories that women seem to fall into when they're pregnant. In fact, scrap the last part of that sentence. Pregnant or not, there are certain women who possess moderation, and will easily adapt their already sensible diets to the new requirements of pregnancy. The follower of this laughable 'add on 500 calories a day' regime will be the woman who always got her school homework in on time. And she probably had the neatest pencil-case too. She probably now possesses a fair amount of camel/buff/biscuit-coloured clothes in her wardrobe, never wears her knickers two days on the trot and has a salad drawer that freakishly contains salad. They are sensible women who have neat highlights in their well-combed hair. Their cars never smell of bacon crisps or dank plimsolls. They get their Christmas cards sent by 12 December.

And then there's the rest of us Neanderthals.

To us, moderation is a bizarre term that is very rarely used in common parlance, a bit like 'fiefdom' or 'sedan chair'. Moderation, biscuit-clothed women tell me, means that you take just the one Meltis Fruit jelly, rather than one of each colour to keep you going until the tray comes round again. Moderation means exercising three times a week rather than doing the London Marathon once, dressed in a chicken costume, and then coming down with chronic bronchitis. Moderation means going to a party and just drinking the two glasses of dry white wine rather than the four pints of cider, two Snowballs, before getting involved in inventing a new cocktail. Moderation is the dry pretzel as opposed to, say, a big fat cheesy Wotsit. Moderation is deathly dull – a very exacting mistress.

I must confess, in the name of impartial reporting, that I've been on a diet of one sort or other for the last fifteen years. It all started when I went to work as an au pair in Italy aged eighteen and fell in love. Not with a rugged Sicilian or a smooth Milanese. Not with a person at all but a place – Pizzeria Asti. I lived next door to it for eleven months of pure, unadulterated bliss. Our relationship became addictive. We were never apart. I was racking up two hot chocolates and pastries for breakfast, a full three-course, leisurely lunch and then, of an evening, pasta, pizza, ice cream and cake – whatever my love-struck haggis of a stomach could take. When I returned to England I was appalled to look in the mirror and find not the little Audrey Hepburn figure who'd pranced off to Italy for her Roman Holiday, but a female version of Sandro Ciotti, the enormous old Italian football commentator, who made John Prescott look handsome.

A strict diet ensued, instigated by my mother. She became the Keeper of the Larder, and patrolled the area with a jar of appetite-suppressing sesame seeds.

The diet she put me on was called the 'I Love Wholemeal! Diet' with that zanily placed exclamation mark to make the whole thing seem a really fun thing to do. You might as well have called it the 'I Love Holidaying With Joseph Stalin Diet'. No one could love it. The whole concept of wholemeal is not lovable. I knuckled under because I had no choice.

So here I am at a crucial fork in the road. In fact, there's not only a large fork, there's a knife, plate and napkin too. On the one side – moderation. This road – seven months of sensible meals – looks bare and bleak, and there are some hunched ramblers far up ahead with spindly little legs. Or I could take the other road – profligacy. A road lined with cafés, restaurants and fast-food outlets. There's a delicious smell emanating from it and ruddy-faced people are having a gay old time. It's all easy-rolling hills and verdant pastures – there are even electric golf-carts so you don't have to use your legs. And look! Isn't that Pizzeria Asti over there in the distance? Its friendly wood-smoke curls out of the chimney and it seems to call out to me, 'Join us! Join the Gorgers, the Slackers, the Porkers! Diet later! Join us!'

There's no question really. Stuff the mealy-mouthed Moderates and stuff me instead! I return to the fridge.

199 days to go ...

I'M TRYING TO BELIEVE THAT yesterday's fridge visit was just a daytrip. I'm not seeking a permanent visa – it was just a one-off, a fly-past. But if I'm being honest I'm ruddy starving. Most people are in the morning, but not if you factor in that I've already had a full cooked breakfast less than an hour ago.

As a delaying tactic I seek counsel with the TV doctor. There's a chapter called 'Essential Nutrition' which could be helpful. It might have some nice winter-warmer type recipes in it, wholesome but filling.

I can't find the book. Dan seems to have moved it again. He's spending a lot of time with his nose in it at the moment – far more than me. I finally find it in Dan's briefcase decorated with Post-Its. One is marking the 'Coping With Fatherhood' chapter and the other is firmly placed on a page headed 'Hormonal Mood Swings'.

I fly to 'Essential Nutrition' in quiet anticipation. My heart sinks. There must be some mistake here. There are pictures of piles of wholegrains, pieces of melon, nuts and seeds, brown pasta. This is the 'I Love Bloody Wholemeal! Diet' all over again. What I see before me on this prim, wholesome, gruesome little page is not enough to keep my guinea-pig alive.

Dan's home from work early and I seek some sympathy. I show him the rotten book.

'Oh yes. Five hundred cals more than you'd normally have per day.'

This is worrying. He has seamlessly shortened the word calories to cals without batting an eyelid. Things take an even worse turn when he continues, 'I've been thinking we could establish a rolling salad bowl. You know, lots of different bits of salad and veg cut into handy chunks every day, so that if you start to get hungry you can dip into it.'

Oh Judas, I will shun your kiss. What has happened to you? Only two days with that bloody book and your mind has been poisoned! Come back to me, come into my flabby arms and let me breathe some Kipling Manor House cake fumes into your face.

I thought he might understand. Perhaps suggest we ring for a curry together. But suddenly Dan seems very unlike Dan. Not like my ally in all this but my enemy and jailer. My jaw opens and shuts in search of a response like a stunned trout, then my bottom lip trembles and it's off to the bedspread I go. Dan doesn't bother responding to the sound of weeping from upstairs any more. He's immune to these outbursts, especially now that he's got his bloody book.

198 days to go ...

No more mention of the rolling salad bowl today, thank goodness. And something happened today which I can really say might be the start of something beautiful.

I was talking at Pawel over a cup of his weak, over-milky tea, when I suddenly felt a buzzing sensation in my upper gums. Itchy, but quite nice. Sort of warm and comforting. It was harmless, really. I had just shaved off a little piece of Cheddar from the block in the fridge and slipped it into my mouth as I was chatting.

Pawel left the house soon after and I cleared up the tea things, but my mind keeps wandering back to the cool interior of the fridge. I open the door and my eye is drawn to the Cheddar again. It looks a mite untidy. I get the knife again and just neaten things up a bit. I take the block to the table and idly pare away at it. Before I know it, I've whittled it down to almost nothing at all. It sits in the pit of my stomach, melting away like a big fondu. I feel at ease, content, a bit cheeky and very, very happy. It's seems pointless leaving what's left, it's so small. So down it goes with the rest.

I ring Dan and ask him to pick up a few bits and bobs on the way home. A newspaper, some bath cleaner, oh and I almost forgot, maybe a bit of Cheddar?

An hour without is enough to refuel my passion. I hear the key in the door and pounce. I take the bag from Dan, empty the contents onto the worktop and dig in straight from the packet. Dan looks on, amazed, perhaps a little disturbed.

'Do you ... would you like me to make you a sandwich with that cheese?'

But his words fall away unheard, I'm lost in my new love. Dan backs out of the kitchen to seek solace in the telly. Once alone I get down to the serious business of cheese osmosis. I hunch over the block and become a one-woman production line. Faf! The Cheddar is sliced. Woof! Into the mouth. Faf! Woof! Faf! Woof! Faf! Woof! And so on until gradually I begin to calm down.

197 days to go ...

WE'VE GOT OUR FIRST SCAN at the hospital tomorrow. I suppose I should say that I'm really excited about it because it will be the first inkling we'll get that there really is a baby 'in there'. But my mind is on other things. I say 'things'. Just the one thing, actually. Cheese.

I am getting selective about my Cheddar. I'm not just going to take anything that's available at the cornershop or supermarket. I don't want goods cut with 90 per cent man-made emulsified dairy solids. I want the good stuff, the pure shit, know what I'm saying? I head into town to a street where I've been told there's a cheese dealer, cheesemonger, sorry, who can satisfy my special needs.

Ah! There it is on the corner – Mistress Liddyard's. I look in through the window like a Dickensian orphan at Christmas time. Rack upon rack of handmade cheese. And inside, a whole shelf which appears to be dedicated just to Cheddar! My salivary glands are already pricking to attention. All of the assistants are in Edwardian-looking aprons and the Cheese Chief – with big whiskers and walrus moustache – has his name-badge proudly emblazoned on his considerable breast: 'Eddie'. My saviour. I leave the shop with a waxy two-pound package bumping comfortably against my thigh.

196 days to go ...

WE DRAW UP OUTSIDE the hospital and my heart sinks. It's a dour Gothic Victorian monstrosity. Forbidding blackened turrets look down with mean windows and a high wall surrounds the entire area.

'You see, this is just typical, Dan. Not only do women have to go through the pain of giving birth but look where they have to do it.'

There are no curtains at the windows, and an eerie silence. No comforting sound of squealing babies, no motherly nurses emerging with reassuring clipboards.

I feel a sudden wave of envy as I consider the kind of swanky places Posh Spice and the like have their babies. This looks like the Hammer House of Horror in comparison. I wouldn't bat an eyelid if Vincent Price walked out in green scrubs with a stethoscope round his neck.

'It's quite bleak,' admits Dan. 'Are you OK to go inside on your own while I find a parking space?'

'I suppose so,' I reply with a sigh that reflects the thousands of years of shared collective pain of womanhood that I alone, of all my sex, have to bear. I lower my shoulders a little as I get out of the car just to enforce the point.

God, this hospital's a dump. No cheery signs, no cheery 'We're the NHS and My God We're Positive!' posters. Even Henry Cooper and his wife advertising flu jabs would be a lightener at this point in time. A huge crow squawks very close by to me, and I practically jump out of my skin. If the outside is as unprepossessing as this, I'm starting to worry about the inside, and more importantly, what kind of equipment they make do with. A Spinning Jenny to power the scanner, one metal birthing stool and an iron maiden for mothers to recover in. The security man lurks in a little booth just outside. It's sad that they have to have so much security in hospitals these days. I smile my most winning television smile and say pleasantly, 'I've got an appointment.'

'Visiting?'

'Yes, I'm not here to stay. Not yet!' I pat my stomach by way of explanation.

'Well, you don't want to stay here, miss.'

'I won't mind the odd night.'

'You would have a very odd night if you stayed in there.'

I am slightly scared now. I whip a little nugget of cheese out of my pocket just to comfort myself.

'Well, where do I have to go?'

'Which wing's he in?'

'Who, the doctor?'

'Who's ill?'

'No, I'm not ill.'

'Is the person you're visiting ill?'

'I'm visiting the doctor.'

'He's not ill as far as I know.'

I am really befuddled now. A sudden wave of tiredness comes over me, with a dash of nausea mixed in for good measure.

'Look,' I say, taking matters in hand, 'I've got my twelve-week scan, where do I go?'

'Oh, you'll want the maternity hospital. Modern building next door.'

'Excuse me?'

'This is Wormwood Scrubs.'

Thank the Lord Sweet Jesus. There is a God somewhere up there, and He has shown me through some nice swishing automatic doors into the cleanest and brightest of places imaginable. The snack machine looks good and creatively stocked, the receptionists are smiley. Good old NHS. My eyes momentarily brim, as I look around at all the bustling people. I'm feeling proud and just a tad smug that we made the decision to go NHS rather than all poncey and private.

I follow the signs and finally arrive at the scan reception desk. The woman on duty looks at me quizzically when I hand her my doctor's referral letter, then a little smile comes over her lips. I know this look of old. It means that she's recognised me from the telly.

'Don't I know you?' she asks.

'Well, I'm not sure,' I say rather coyly, going into well-trodden banter here. 'Either I'm a long-lost relative of yours, or you might have seen me on your small screen, when I was—'

'It's Mel, isn't it?'

'That's right!'

'I've never seen you on the telly. We waitressed at the same restaurant. L'Express? You were on the griddle.'

Dan arrives at this point having parked the car. He is practically exploding with mirth.

'Wormwood Scrubs, eh?' he guffaws.

I give him a hard stare and turn again to the receptionist. 'L'Express? Yeah, I did waitress there, it was years ago.'

'Well, I never forget a face.'

'I'm really sorry. I'm terrible with names – what's yours?'

'Kelly.'

'Oh hi, Kelly. This is my husband Dan. We've got a twelve-week scan appointment.'

'OK, I'll just check you on the list.'

Dan can hardly contain himself. 'So they didn't keep you in then?'

'Ha ha ha.'

I'm feeling grouchy now. I desperately need to rest my pins.

Then Kelly pipes up. 'So, Mel, what are you up to now? Are you still waitressing?'

I feel the whole left side of my face clench and my cheekbone twitches. 'No, Kelly. I'm actually a broadcaster.'

How the hell did *that* word come out of my mouth? Broadcaster?

'Oh right,' Kelly says. 'Is that, like, on a ship or something?'

We're in a darkened room. It all feels a bit *Starship Enterprise*, quite relaxing. Hi-tech machinery bleeps comfortingly. Suddenly I feel the pressure's off. Somebody else can take control of my baby for a while. I'm lying with my waistband rolled down to reveal my cottage loaf of a stomach. And it's a cottage loaf before it's been baked – a huge swirl of white dough with a horrible crusty belly-button in the middle. Sandra, the nice scan lady, has a weird gearstick thing and she puts some very cold clear jelly all over my loaf. Yikes!

'OK, just relax, we'll just move this around over your tummy and see what we can see.'

Well, there's nothing at the moment, just a tuned-out screen with lots of black fuzz on it. Oh God, maybe it's all been a mistake. It does happen. I'll be one of those poor women who can never have a baby and push dolls around in pushchairs. Dan squeezes my hand reassuringly and Sandra presses the gearstick down rather worryingly on what may be my bladder. Then suddenly we see it. But it's not a baby. No, it's a little astronaut. It's like that blurry black-and-white footage of Buzz Aldrin landing on the moon. It's incredible! It's floating around in there like a little man in a suit! It's kind of hilarious, like an animation of something. It's so alive and so ... uh-oh, here come the waterworks. I look at Dan and he's a goner too. His jaw is shaking and his eyes are brimful. Sandra looks on benignly. Poor thing must have seen this thousands of times.

'It's ... it's our baby!'

'Ye-e-e-s,' she says.

'And I thought I'd just see piles of cheese in there!'

'It looks human enough to me. You see its wee head just there? And there are its legs and arms.'

'Oh my God, it's so beautiful!'

'It's quite lively, it's moving around a lot.'

'Oh, that's so me. Always on the go. Oh look, Dan, it's waving at us! It just waved! Did you see?'

Sandra wisely decides to ignore this. 'I'll get you a printout, shall I?'

'Oh yes, yes! Thank you!'

We can't help poring and poring over the photo of our baby.

'It's definitely got the Parkinson brow,' says Dan, referring to his mum's side of the family. 'Look at that frown.'

'That's not a frown, that's concentration. I can already tell that he or she is very advanced. It's got focus and preparation. And, oh my God, Dan, did you see when it waved at us?'

'No, I didn't see that, but wasn't the break-dancing amazing? And when it did the handjiving, wasn't that great?'

I punch Dan a little bit too hard in the crown jewels for that last comment. And I make him stop at the cheese shop on the way home.

195 days to go ...

ONE OF MY KEY PREGNANCY promises has been broken already. The scan photo has been mounted in a tiny silver frame above the mantelpiece.

192 days to go ...

PICKED UP A MESSAGE from mum on the answerphone today: 'Darling, thanks ever so for the scan picture. Not sure if you've seen, but I'm sure I can make out Baby sucking its thumb. You don't want the little thing to get into bad habits so early. See what you can do.'

189 days to go ...

I CAN'T STOP THINKING OF Mistress Liddyard's. I dropped in again this morning and then felt anxious that I'd under-bought. It finally got too much for me and I went back in the afternoon pretending that I had forgotten something specific to a recipe, which happened to be a block of organic Welsh Cheddar.

188 days to go ...

I REALLY DIDN'T MEAN TO DO IT, I think I was a bit frazzled, but I called Dan 'Eddie' by mistake. He was a bit upset and kept asking me who 'Eddie' was. I blamed it on my hormones. Rather than coming clean and saying that Eddie is a cheesemonger around the age of sixty-five with an enormous paunch and gin blossoms on his face, I said nothing. I want to keep my secret cheese life to myself.

187 days to go ...

TRIED A PIECE OF alderwood smoked Cheddar today. Quite nice and smoky, but a little too showy. I now carry a little Tupperware box around with me in my bag, with pre-cut slices of cheese, so that I don't have to mess around with knives. People can get the wrong idea if you pull a knife out on public transport.

186 days to go ...

I WONDER IF I'm going to have any cravings during this pregnancy?

185 days to go ...

I ASKED DAN that very same question today. He spat out his coffee rather too close to my face, and laughed in a rather brittle way.

'Of course you've got a craving, you fool. Anyway, why ask me? Why don't you go and ask your lover, whassisname Eddie?'

'Well, I think Eddie probably has some idea that I like cheese ... He's a cheesemonger ... at Mistress Liddyard's.' My head is bowed, I can feel my cheeks going hot with shame.

Dan looks stunned and then throws his head back and laughs and laughs, and does that silly thing that men do when they laugh too much, which is to clutch his own plums.

I knew I shouldn't have told him about Eddie. I'm never going to hear the end of this now.

180 days to go ...

GUILT HAS FINALLY GOT the better of me more than three weeks after receiving Amanda's message. I phone her.

'Hello! You've reached Amanda and Roger's answer-machine. We're not here but do leave a message, or try us in Majorca (long number). Or try our mobes (more long numbers). Bye.'

I don't think I've ever heard such a smug answerphone message. Why am I friends with this woman? It rubbed me up the wrong way and I must have sounded as if I'd just swallowed a spoonful of vinegar as I left my message.

'Amanda, have you had it yet? Call me. It's Mel.'

Actually my sister Kate's message would push her pretty hard. It says: 'Hi, if you'd like to leave a message for Kate, Jake, Tom or Jessica, please speak after the tone.'

Now, hang on. Tom is four, Jessica nearly two. Why the hell would I want to leave them a message? To arrange to meet them for a drink? I'm afraid simple smugness is the answer here – they are merely displaying to the world that they have not one but *two* children and aren't they clever? Dan and I will never leave a recorded message like that on our answerphone.

My 'mobe' rings. I pick it up and there's a lot of heavy breathing followed by a thick Leeds-accented voice saying, 'Hello, Mel, it's Eddie. I think you look very GOUDA at the moment. Would you BRIE available to come out on a date? I'm very MATURE...' And then gales of wheezing laughter. I bet Dan took about half an hour to think that up.

175 days to go …

I KEEP WANDERING INTO Pawel's room and imagining all of the groovy things I'm going to do with it when he's gone. A little mural of a farm here, a nightlight there. Some nice Babar the elephant curtains perhaps. It's hard to visualise all this right now. Pawel's room is crammed, ceiling to floor, with old brown files with indecipherable things written on the sides. I've never known a language with so many Zs in it. He sounds like a little wasp when you hear him on the phone back to his family in Warsaw. Bzz pzzzszz crzz.

As I dream of the perfect nursery, surrounded by Pawel's rather antiquated stationery and his framed picture of the Pope, I make the momentarily shocking discovery of a porn mag peeking out from under his mattress. On closer inspection it is just one volume – called *Juggs*, for the record – of a rather extensive collection. As a landlady and mother-to-be, I'm feeling slightly sullied and ever more eager to get my new broom to work in here.

170 days to go ...

LAST NIGHT I HAD the most appalling cheese-induced rollercoaster of a nightmare. I dreamt of Eddie. But it was no longer affable Eddie in his endearing stripy apron. This was Eddie as a sort of Jeff Stryker figure – in black leather chaps and a bandanna round his neck. His bare chest was oiled and his lips strangely moist. The nightmare was set to a heavy electro-funk beat. Mistress Liddyard's had been transformed into a dry-ice-filled den of vice, with assistants lolling around in knickers on the counters looking moody with tongues hanging out. Very distressing. I looked down to see that I was wearing a pink fluffy negligee, handcuffs and a pair of navy deck shoes. And I was mewling. Then Eddie led me over to the Cheddar section and every cheese was dripping – it was like a big sex fondue.

'Oh Eddie!' I barely recognised my own voice – I sounded like Rula Lenska. 'Eddie – please give me a big knob.'

'You're going to have to beg me for it, honey.'

Hang on a second, Eddie was suddenly speaking in a Texan accent. He's from Ilkley!

'Oh please, Eddie, you know I need a big knob every six hours.'

'Well OK, sugar, but only cos Eddie knows you've been a good little kitty. I'm gonna give it to you right now.'

And with that Eddie minces over to the cheese-cutter, revealing a pair of calves like upturned magnums of champagne and ... oh my goodness me, sock suspenders! His whiskers are moist, he leers at me through half-closed eyes and brings the cheese wire down tantalisingly just so that it's resting on the top of the Cheddar.

'Oh yes, Eddie!' I'm helpless, panting and whispering like Marilyn Monroe at President Kennedy's birthday party. 'Oh Eddie, make it a big one. A super big one. You know I can take it.'

Eddie has turned me into a Cheese Whore. Before long I'll be standing outside all the cheesemongers of London selling my own curds and whey. Oh God, Eddie's my pimp and I'll be his spotty, overweight mess of a prostitute. I'll give birth to a baby addict who needs to be fed Red Leicester every two hours like its mother. How can I break the cycle? Eddie bears down on me like an enormous sea-lion … he is offering me cheese from his own rank-smelling tongue … I am just about to take both the cheese and his liverish tongue into my own mouth when …

Phew! All is as it should be. Dan snoring gently beside me. My cheese by the bed in its normal place. I ponder this cheese insanity with the cheesy porn soundtrack still ringing in my ears. This is craven behaviour.

I lie there pondering the varying degrees of craven manifested during pregnancy.

There's the Gemma Craven. She is the pregnant lady who'll have a craving for something like lime cordial or oatcakes. She'll sip and peck at her snacks like a dainty little bumble-bee.

Then there are the John Cravens. Their appetite is a little more male and hearty than the Gemmas. They'll probably crave pasties and sausages and don't mind wolfing the goods in front of other people.

Then there is the last and very special category of Cravens. I count myself among their number. Welcome to the Wes Cravens. We are the wild-eyed bunch of pregnant women with scary Freddie Kruger knife-fingers who will prong anything in their sights. Be it Cheddar, cake, canapés, gherkins, quiche or Scotch eggs. Keep foodstuffs in your house at your own peril when there's a Wes in the area – we will eat you out of house, home and we'll eat your children too if we can find the right condiment. Oh God, I must do some exercise or I'm going to be as big as my Auntie Ursula who ate so much during her pregnancies she had to sit on a reinforced chair like the Queen of Tonga.

165 days to go ...

I SPOKE TO AMANDA TODAY. For once I actually picked up the phone without screening and the old goat managed to annoy me within about two seconds.

The thing about being pregnant is that you and only you are the epicentre of the universe for that nine months, and nobody else can be allowed to take that away from you. So if you have a friend who is pregnant at the same time as you, you would be well advised to avoid them like the plague. Do you want someone capping your Hilarious Cravings Anecdote with something even funnier? Do you want them pulling the ill-informed medical rug from under you? Do you want to hear someone else's whingeing morning sickness stories? No. Your pregnancy gives you the watertight excuse to take a long swim in Lake You. Make the most of it. Two pregnant women in a confined space might cause a loud whining.

'Hi, Mel. God! I'm about to drop, but I'm feeling absolutely fabby. How are you?'

She's been saying fabby since the eighties. Is it just a bad line or can I hear the hormonal feedback starting to whine already?

'Well, let's put it this way, I haven't quite reached that heady bloom stage. In fact, I've been feeling pretty grim – like I'm in a bath and my plug's been pulled, draining me of all my water.'

In the middle of my heartfelt speech I become aware that Amanda is tapping away on her computer. Lightly, deftly – her French-polished talons rattling over the keyboard. I want to hang up on her, but the old power hold gets the better of me and I simply peter to an apologetic halt.

'Look, Mel babes, why don't you swing by tomorrow morning? I'll fix us something nice and we can swap stories. Are you doing lots of exercise?'

164 days to go ...

I ASCEND THE STEPS TO Amanda's house with heavy feet and heart and brace myself. Before I even get a chance to knock, she opens the door and swings her luxuriant honey mane of hair in a single studied movement.

'Mel!'

She smells spriggy and lineny as I kiss her. She is tanned and wearing stilettos and suede trousers with the waistband under ... the bitch ... yes, ***under*** her perfect, high, neat, tight bump. The look is completed with a crisp white cotton shirt and lots of undoubtedly expensive and rather aggressive-looking jewellery. If she threw her necklace like a Frisbee, it'd decapitate you. It pains me to admit, but she actually looks much sexier pregnant. The horsier features of her face have softened, her usually David Bowie-esque teeth look somehow less sharky and goddammit she doesn't seem to have put on an ounce, bar the bump, of course.

I am wearing my usual grubby hi-top trainers, jeans which bulge so much at the top that I now have to open two of the fly buttons, an old tie-dye shirt and rather too many clips in my hair in an attempt to compensate for an overall lack of styling. I have bags, I have jowls, I have crevices. I look like a championship snooker player. Amanda imperceptibly shakes her head.

'Babe, come on in! I've juiced us up some nice light vegetables. Fancy a spritzer-juice or just as it comes?'

'Got any custard creams?'

She forces a laugh. 'Mel, you haven't changed. Still crazy about ... what were those things we used to eat at your house? Jammy Dodgers. Eurgh!'

'Well, what's this then?' I say, eyeing the bleak-looking contents of Amanda's perfect hi-ball glass. 'Looks like the by-product of a colonic irrigation.'

'Beanshoot, ginseng and carrot.'

She whizzes me up a fresh batch with an awkward smile. I try to do better.

'So how are you, Amanda? It's been ages.'

'Mel, I feel brilliant. Honestly. Isn't it just the best thing being pregnant? I never realised! It's just so … so sexy and wonderful.'

'Any nausea? Any cravings?'

'Yes! I had the most bizarre craving ever. Lettuce! Isn't that hysterical? And not just any lettuce. Had to be Cos. Only Cos. PLATEFULS of the stuff! I look like Bugs Bunny. Munch, munch! What about you? You look like you've had some cravings!'

My jaw tightens. I count to ten as Amanda breezes on, 'Yes, Kate got very porky when she was pregnant.'

I know 'Kate' must be a celebrity, but I'm damned if I'm going to give Amanda the satisfaction of asking her which Kate.

'Well, it's lovely to see you. Now you've GOT to see the nursery. Come on, bring your juice.'

As we pass a big silver tray hanging in the Indian-themed hallway, I catch an unwelcome sight of myself. These past weeks have caught up with me. I now realise, seeing Amanda, that Dan's been soft-soaping me. We shimmy over parquet floors, until Amanda throws open the door on to a room bigger than our lounge.

'Well? What do you think? They finished it yesterday.'

'They', whoever they are, have certainly done an interesting job. I stare open-mouthed around me.

'It's very … er … contemporary,' I say in the end. 'Has a certain Damien Hirst feel to it.'

The flooring is made entirely of soft leather, apart from one rug, which, as a concession to the child, has a cartoon baby saying 'Wah!' on it. Very Lichtenstein. And there are lots of vases filled with twigs everywhere. Hard to pin a theme on this room. The crib, if it is a crib, looks custom-built out of, I think, stainless steel.

'It doesn't rock,' Amanda explains. 'Rocking can make the baby feel claustrophobic. It slides to and fro on castors – see!'

It's a bit like keeping your baby in a filing cabinet.

'Tommy created it for me, you remember Tommy my fabby designer friend. He's so clever!'

There are Perspex shelves from floor to ceiling containing every item of clothing that you can possibly imagine a baby might need – mini-puffa jackets, fleeces, diddy cashmere sweaters, little Gucci shoes and, I swear, a tiny Louis Vuitton grip-bag.

'For weekends away?'

'For skiing,' Amanda replies, without irony. You couldn't make it up.

'Skiing?'

'Oh yes, they can start when they're practically still in arms.'

'How exactly?' I'm genuinely intrigued now, imagining little knitted skis and poles.

'Oh, you attach them to one ski and kind of drag them down the slope, I think.'

'Amanda, you are joking. Drag a baby down the slope? On one ski?'

'That's what my instructor tells me, yeah.'

'I don't know if they have Social Services in Val d'Isère but if they do they'll be on to you in a nano second!'

'Not Val d'Isère, Mel.' She wrinkles her nose. 'That's for the shell-suit brigade. Whistler is the place – you and Dan must try it once we've both got this horrible business out of the way!'

And with that the subject is closed. This is typical Amanda. Wave the problem away with a manicured hand. Don't analyse, just do. Babies can ski. They will ski, that's that. You can pay people to organise it.

My eye is caught by a spacious walnut bookshelf. Amanda's filled it with every conceivable Beatrix Potter book – get this – in English, French and Italian!

'*Pierre Lapin et Monsieur Macgregor? La Signora Tiggywinkle?*'

'I want it to grow up multi-lingual. Look how it's helped Princess Stephanie of Monaco.'

I suddenly start to feel a bit sorry for poor little It. And perhaps a little bit for myself too. I suddenly have a real pang to be back home, in our small, slightly grubby, non-event of a flat.

'You leave nothing to chance,' is the best I can do without offending her. 'I really should get going soon, I've got to do a big shop.'

'Shouldn't Dan do that? You look ever so peaky, Mel. My yoga teacher's coming in a sec and you could do some relaxation with us. I can lend you slacks and a mat.'

'You're very sweet, Amanda, but I'd better make tracks. Thanks for showing me round. How's Roger by the way?'

A slight shadow passes over her face. 'Oh. He's in Portugal at the mo. Hopes to have things tied up and be back in a week or so.'

I now feel rather sorry for her. 'Well, let us know if you need anything.'

'Oh God, I'm fine. Everything under control. I've even got my bag packed to take to the hospital. Do you want to have a look?'

'I must be off. Thanks for the lovely juice.'

We embrace in a slightly awkward way, Amanda trying to avoid my greasy, clip-filled hair.

'Well, get Roger to phone us when anything happens. Two weeks left! Blimey. Good luck.'

'I'm looking forward to it all being over. I just want to start my circuit training and boxercise again.'

160 days to go ...

SPOKE BRIEFLY TO MUM on the phone today. Her parting shot was, 'Darling, I was reading in one of those magazines today that the doctors think Baby can hear everything you say, even though it's inside. You and Dan must keep your swearing and all that modern talk down to a minimum. If you put your mind to it, you could even start repeating the useful phrases it will need for good company: "please", "thank you", "may I get down from the table?" that kind of thing. Nothing like a head start – manners still maketh man.'

154 days to go ...

I START THE *EX MANIAC* PRE-PRODUCTION tomorrow and have begun to panic that I've nothing to wear at all. Having abandoned the Get Rid of the Navy project all those weeks ago, my wardrobe is still in a pretty sorry state. I decide to put things into piles. This is a great technique for not actually throwing anything away at all. I split my clothes into two piles: stuff that I can carry on wearing and stuff that I can't. I'm being brutal and so the latter forms a tottering tower of pretty much everything I own, while the other is barely a pile: two pairs of trousers (one drawstring and the other elasticated) and a couple of T-shirts that I only wear to sleep in. One has a Monet print on it and the other says 'Women Are Angry'.

Oh God. How do people like bloody Amanda manage to look so damn good while being pregnant? The sensible TV lady doctor's pregnancy book is not much help either. There are loads of photos of couples in freakishly matching outfits. The man is always standing behind the woman with his arms encircling her, hands intertwined and resting lightly on the Bump. The woman stretches her neck back to look lovingly at him. She wears a lavender blue smock with matching accessories and he has lavender slacks and a rather daring lemon aertex shirt. On another page they're there again indulging in some couple-oriented light relaxation together. She hugs a mug of some hot herbal beverage and he jokily tries to feed her a beanshoot. She's now gone casual in puce dungarees with little lavender socklets, and he sports a pair of loose jeans and a lemon rugby shirt. Much more frightening is the final picture of her in a lavender jumpsuit with horrible spongy epaulettes and oversized buttons.

I can see what the sensible lady doctor's trying to do here. She's trying to turn all of us expectant mothers into babies! That lavender jumpsuit is basically an adult-sized babygro. How grim, and how humiliating. I will not succumb to the babygro! Even if I expand to the size of Demis Roussos. I would rather go naked and only move around under cover of darkness.

I need help. I ring the show's producer in a bit of a paddy and she calmly arranges for me to go shopping with the costume lady tomorrow.

153 days to go ...

I MEET SARAH, the costume lady, outside Oxford Circus tube station. Everything seems frantic, loud and manic. It makes me realise what a recluse I've become these last few months. I actually haven't been anywhere near the West End since I found out I was pregnant. I feel like a bumpkin who's just arrived in town from Shropshire with a stick and bundle. And what's chic seems to have changed since I last took an interest. Everyone that passes, the women anyway, are in the tiniest of mini-skirts, floppy gypsy-like tops and strange stiletto shoes with socks on. And everyone's gone a strange colour! They all look really orange and a bit shiny.

'It's the Costa del Sol sun-kissed trash look,' Sarah informs me.

'Well, I'm sure I could fit into one of those floppy top-things. My rack has expanded by at least two cup sizes already!'

I'm glad of the imminent attention and pampering, and feel full of verve and enthusiasm. Sarah ushers me into the first changing room with my arms piled high with gypsy tops, micro-skirts, stringy vests, hipster trousers and off-the-shoulder sweat-tops. I'm determined to cut a sartorial dash on this show.

I reach for a size 14 floppy top and can barely get my shoulder through the hole. Once it's kind of on, I look like an enormous homemade cream cheese that is groaning and dripping through a muslin sack. I approach the mini-skirt like a nervous horse at Beecher's Brook. No, no way. I am surrounded on all sides by younger, thinner, less pregnant women. I feel out of touch, lumbering, useless, old and suddenly utterly exhausted. The music's too loud and the heat is pumped right up in these high street chain shops. And there are too many people. A girl in crop top and roller-skates shrieks into her mobile phone and jolts me as she flies out of the shop. I am forced sharply into a stand of fluffy handcuffs. I have become middle-aged. I don't fit in! I'm an alien! Return me back to Planet Hatchback! Right there, in the middle of the shop floor, I cry lustily. Poor old Sarah, she's only just met me and here I am sobbing in her arms like an emotionally incontinent lunatic.

'I want to go home,' I sob, like a three-year-old who's been bullied at a party.

Sarah lightly manoeuvres me out of the shop and into a cab home. I am completely shredded. I take to my bed for the rest of the day with a family bag of prawn cocktail crisps and a jar of beetroot.

152 days to go ...

SARAH THE COSTUME LADY has come good. She has abandoned Costa del Sol for the Floppy Surrey look, thank God. She's bought me a range of clothes which are lightweight, loose-fitting, and mercifully nothing in lavender. They tend towards the dark end of the spectrum – long skirts cut on the bias, roomy tops with cunning accessories (a fake magnolia, a rococo brooch) to divert attention from the enormous Galia melons residing in my bra. And crucially, an item of clothing which must signify that I have come of age: Sarah has bought me 'palazzo pants'. Elaine Paige wears them. They are a loose, show-business trouser with an 'easy kick' and a 'long ride' (i.e. they hide chunky calves and don't cling round your nethers). They are fabulously comfortable and I want to cry with relief in Sarah's arms. Thankfully I resist, because that would mean a 100 per cent blubber-rate since I met her. I don't want her to think that I'm mentally unstable. My friends must never ever see me in the palazzo pants. If they even catch a whiff of their billowing flare in my wardrobe, I'm done for.

I twirl in front of a long mirror and feel pretty good for the first time in ages. I still look like a matriarchal folk singer from certain angles – you might catch me at the Cropredy Festival singing 'My Lady D'Arbanville' – but I'd rather that than look like a tubby wannabe who's gone beyond mutton dressed as lamb into the whole new dimension of gammon dressed as spam.

It gives me just the confidence I need, as today I must rediscover the Media Ballbreaker within. I'm determined to stride into our initial production meeting with a swing in my palazzo pants, to show these TV people that I'm not just Rent-a-Presenter.

The meeting is in the offices of Duchess TV Productions. We sit round a glass table in a rather stifling boardroom. The lift is out of order and my struggle up three flights of stairs has given me a moustache of sweat, which I feel pricking under my nostrils. Coffee and tea are brought round and a large plateful of luxury biscuits – no thanks! Just a simple black coffee for the Media Ballbreaker this morning!

Lucinda McCleod chairs the meeting – she's a fifty-something TV exec who's been in the biz pretty much since there was one very crackly channel. She invented *Nationwide* and was personally responsible for discovering Frank Bough. She has a Great Dane called Hamlet who lies at her feet. Everything about her is spiky, from her heels to her earrings, cheekbones and silly handbag. She starts to address the gathering, consisting mainly of twenty-something eager beavers, who hunch over their notes, drinking in every word she says, as if she were the Delphic oracle. She opens her scarlet spiky mouth and doesn't draw breath for at least twenty minutes – 'audience share', 'programme remit', 'B/C Group', 'Neo-Reality TV' and so it continues.

My eye is caught by a lovely fig tree in the corner of the room. Somebody has taken care to buff each of its leaves individually so that they shine like lilypads on a pond. It is only one plant yet it manages to spring forth from its pot like a corps de ballet. I wonder how often it needs watering. Is it possible to get actual figs from an indoor plant like this? I must ask at my local garden centre. How wonderful nature is! How clever, how simple, yet how indescribably complicated the whole system—

'Mel?'

Every pair of eyes looks at me expectantly. Lucinda's glower over her glasses like my geography teacher's used to.

'Yes?' I say lamely.

'We were just wondering what your view is on how we innovate the reality element of *Ex Maniac*?'

My sweat moustache pricks up again and I can feel my armpits following suit. Come on, Mel. Break some balls. Say something pithy.

'Yeah, absolutely, for me the reality aspect is very much the essence of the show and er ... It's what gives it cutting edge and we need to innovate or perish. Perhaps we could workshop it through?'

There is a silence round the table. One researcher smiles at me patronisingly.

'Anything else?' asks Lucinda.

Even Hamlet's giving me the gimlet eye.

'I don't suppose anyone knows if that fig tree's a fruit-producer?'

And with that my hand goes out to the plate and I sink my teeth into a luxury biscuit.

151 days to go ...

TODAY THE REAL WORK STARTS. After yesterday's sorry attempts to cut it as a media-savvy chick I think that the best policy is to keep as low a profile as possible. I will be Workhorse Presenter today. Low-key, ever vigilant and very, very friendly with everyone. You know what they say – be nice to the lowest person on the crew because one day they could be director-general of the BBC. I decide to focus my attention on a boy called Lucas who seems to be running around a lot. We're in a shopping centre in Lewisham. The production design team have erected a secret booth in which a hand-picked divorcee and I will sit, unseen, and basically spy on people. The air is filled with pomposity. Researchers, assistant producers and everyone else talks a lot of nonsense into walkie-talkies as if they're on an SAS mission: 'Hi Sebastian? Yah, Henrietta here. Just coming upstairs with the release form. Over and out.'

Once we actually start filming, the divorcee will then spy on lots of people in the shopping centre and choose an unlikely person for a date, a person who is the polar opposite to his or her ex. Simple.

I ask Lucas where he's from, laugh at his anecdotes and cajole him into telling me about his love life. It's only when someone tells him he's needed back at Hornes Menswear, that I realise he works at the shopping centre and is nothing at all to do with TV. I shun him immediately and am mortified by my own shallowness.

We spend the day walking through the basic outline of the show. I grab two hours of kip on a stockroom floor and am given a whole wad of research notes on tomorrow's divorcee who's called Michelle. Then there are protracted goodbyes involving lots of hugs to all members of the crew who I've only just met. I can hardly remember most of their names – thus the beauty in television of calling everyone 'my love', 'babe' or 'darling'. Then it's hometime in a nice Merc courtesy of Duchess. What a piece of cake this gig's going to be.

150 days to go ...

I'M WITH MICHELLE, a forty-something, divorcee bingo-caller from Dagenham. I pride myself on having cultivated a rather winning way with members of the public, but once cooped up with this Essex Amazon in the secret *Ex Maniac* booth, I realise that I'm going to have to dig deep into my professional resources.

She eyes me suspiciously under her dry, tight perm. 'So what are you doing on this show then?'

'I'm presenting it.'

'How come you got to be a TV presenter then?'

The same way you got to be a bingo-caller, is the first reply that comes to mind, but my middle-class politeness rears its annoying head in the nick of time.

'Oh, you know, Michelle, the right place at the right time.'

She scratches her perm, so that her mottled upper arm flaps about.

'You've put on a bit of weight, haven't you, Sue?'

'It's Mel. And yes, I have. I'm pregnant.'

'Oh yeah? I've got five of the little bastards and they're all useless.'

You can't really respond to that. I develop an instant and hormonal hatred of her.

Michelle is soaked to the gills in a very strong perfume. It's powerfully reminiscent of the minicab driver's smelly tree and I feel that old familiar saliva start to bubble in my mouth. Oh God, think of something else, I just mustn't be sick. I try discreetly to pull my top up over my nose to block the fumes, but the director keeps signalling me to stop covering my face. I manage to get through an hour of this while Michelle surveys the shopping centre via the web of hidden cameras and lays into the men on offer.

'Look at him, bag of hammers!'

'I've seen more hair on my pitbull's balls!'

'Wanker.'

Then disaster. She takes out the offending bottle of market-stall musk and sprays her hair and underarms. I can wait no longer. I leave the booth and vomit profusely into a nearby yukka.

Henrietta is immediately at my side, proffering a paper hanky. She's a jolly hockey-sticks runner, fresh out of Roedean, and is responsible for predicting and taking care of my every whim. She has obviously tried to fit in with the other trendies at Duchess, but has got it slightly wrong. She is a bit too fat and spotty to carry off the crop top with 'Slag' emblazoned upon it.

'Oh my GOD, Mel, you poor thing. Are you SURE you're all right?'

'Don't worry about me, I'll go back in there and carry on filming!'

The production team encircle me like a legion of worker ants. I feel that they look on me as their selfless leader who alone can sustain our endeavour. At times like these, I must admit, it's really cool being pregnant. People think you're terribly terribly brave for doing absolutely bugger all.

We film for four more long hours. Michelle calls me Sue several hundred times and sprays herself thrice more before we finally find her a bloke and can call it a day. In accordance with the rules of the show, the date must be as different from her ex as is humanly possible. The poor victim she chooses is a nineteen-year-old Swedish backpacker called Klars. He agrees to go on a date with Michelle solely because he'll be paid a hundred quid to do it. He desperately needs the money to get back to Stockholm to see his mother.

149 days to go ...

WE'RE FILMING IN BRIGHTON and today's divorcee is Adam. Adam works in IT and his mouth is so dry the corners of it have collected a white film. His breath is hideous and has a plasticky odour like a new piece of luggage. Miraculously he pulls quite quickly, and I'm not sick, so quite a good day all in all.

148 days to go ...

SUDDENLY IT'S HEATWAVE BRITAIN. The temperature outside is about eighty-five. We're in Ipswich and I have never felt so ill in all my life. My make-up is sliding off my face like a Dali clock and my brain feels like it's been diced, fried and made into jumbalaya. Worst of all, I am stuck in this sweltering bloody booth with the *jolliest* person in the whole of the United Kingdom.

I try to summon up a professional smile for her. 'So, Lucy, where are you from?'

Lucy roars with laughter as if I have just made the most hilarious joke of all time.

'I'm from Ipswich itself,' she manages to say, before peal upon peal of high-pitched laughter ensue.

'I've never really been to Ipswich before, except for when I was a very small child,' I venture, by way of conversation.

Lucy thinks this is the funniest thing she's ever heard, and begins to roll around in her chair and wipe her eyes with a hanky.

'Have you seen anyone you might fancy asking for a date yet?' I ask, trying to calm her down.

Lucy cannot respond. She is laughing so much a glass of water has to be fetched for her.

147 days to go ...

TODAY WE'RE IN NEWCASTLE. The infernal heat shows no sign of abating and hysterical headlines abound: 'NO DROUGHT ABOUT IT – THERE'S A HEATWAVE!' and in London Dan tells me, 'MARBLE PARCH' is the *Evening Standard* headline.

It's not much fun being pregnant in this heat. I just hope the baby's OK. All I want to do is lie in a bath of tepid water with a never-ending supply of cold, sugary drinks to hand. Instead I am in this scorching tardis, in the company of a deaf septuagenarian called Joan who has very little idea or interest in how the show works.

'SO CAN YOU SEE ANYONE NICE, JOAN?'

'Yes, dear. It's very nice.'

'YES, BUT CAN YOU SEE ANYONE YOU MIGHT LIKE TO ASK FOR A DATE, JOAN?'

'Ooh, I don't know about that, dear.'

'WHO DO YOU FANCY, JOAN?'

'I always had a bit of a thing for Bud Flanagan, dear.'

'GREAT! SO HAVE YOU SEEN ANY BUD FLANAGANS HERE?'

'No, I didn't see him here, pet, I saw him before the war. At the Theatre Royal. He's dead now.'

146 days to go ...

It's my day off. Thank goodness. An enormous bunch of flowers consisting mainly of twigs arrives to congratulate me on our first five wonderful days together: 'To Mel. A real trouper! Love, everyone at Duchess.' How ludicrous. How TV. Nevertheless I leave the little card ostentatiously on the kitchen table. I want Dan to think that I've been through the mill, then hopefully he'll do all the cooking and shopping this weekend.

I feel ram-raided, steam-rollered and minced with tiredness and can barely summon the energy for polite conversation. The heat has lessened only to be replaced with Thunder Britain. Dan won't let me go out of the flat because he's worried about the baby being hit by lightning. No mention of me. After the last few days of being treated like a portion of boil-in-the-bag rice, the poor little mite probably wouldn't be troubled by a large crack of lightning, but Dan is adamant.

We're staying in today to tackle the problem areas in the flat. Pinpoint those hazardous child-unfriendly zones that we need to deal with before the baby arrives.

We start with the living room, a key battle area. If you've ever been to an old Russian lady's house you may notice that they love ornaments and favour busy furnishings. I'm afraid to say, I'm something of a West London Babushka. As we scan the scene critically, I realise every available surface is covered with a trinket, knick-knack, keepsake or gew-gaw. I may be only thirty-three but I have no shame in saying that I like a doily. I like little vases and pots, glass animals, postcards, silly homemade things, wooden eggs. My pride and joy though, the pièce de resistance, is my childhood collection of Whimsies. Whimsies were, to my childhood mind, the outstanding invention of the era – an amazing array of china animals that used to come in cute little boxes. Each one cost about two weeks' pocket money and we all used to collect them fanatically at school. I have fifty-eight Whimsies and they are all proudly on display on one of our bookshelves. The boxes that they came in are kept on the shelf below that. Dan has attempted to do away with the Whimsy collection for as long as we've been together, even resorting at one point to smuggling one Whimsy out of the house every day. He presumed I wouldn't notice if the cat with the little pink ball of wool, which sat fifth from the right behind the hippo, disappeared.

Dan's brows are knotted and he sighs deeply.

'Well, that Whimsy collection's got to go for starters.'

'No way.'

'Mel, the baby could easily choke on them.'

'We'll just put them on a higher shelf.'

'OK, what about that clay piece of rubbish?'

'That's a Christmas nest. Little Tom made it for us.'

'What about these bells?'

'They're from India, Pen gave them to me. We can hang them slightly higher up, out of harm's way.'

I suddenly realise there isn't anything in the room that actually belongs to Dan. Apart from a car manual and a Zippo lighter. Men are funny like that. If Dan had his way we'd live on the set of an Ibsen play – bare boards, one chair and one candle. He looks over at my plant collection with the air of a loss adjuster. It's starting to grate on my nerves.

'What about that malodorous plant collection?'

'No way. Each plant is very special to me. Sue's mum gave me the lemon geranium, my mum gave me the spider plants when I first went to college, the yukka's from—'

'Have you any idea just how poisonous some of these plants could be to a baby? It just has to suck on one tiny leaf and—'

'Well, we'll just have to put them out of reach.'

This is rapidly becoming my pat solution to everything I can't bring myself to chuck, which is … well, just about everything.

The colour suddenly drains from my face.

Dan looks alarmed. 'Hey what's up?'

'Look at the windows! Dan, look at them, they're so low. Oh my God! We're going to have to get them heightened.'

'It's OK, we'll just have to make sure the little one doesn't get too close to them once he or she's starting to walk.'

'Dan, we need to talk to a builder now. Look at them. That's insane! They're lower than my waist.'

'I think you might be exaggerating this, Mel.'

'Look, picture the scene: we go to the panto at Christmas. It's *Peter Pan*. We come back. The child thinks it can fly. It opens the window and woosh!'

'Well, we'll make sure we go and see *Jack and the Beanstalk* then.'

'That's worse! It might attempt to shin up the wisteria and then crash! Oh my God, this is terrible. Everything's a hazard. It could lose a whole hand in the ice crusher, it could suffocate in one of the bean-bags.'

Dan physically manoeuvres me up to bed. He reckons I've overdone it this week with the filming. He fetches me a glass of cold water and gently strokes my head.

'What about our bikes in the hallway?'

'Ssshh.'

'And the loo! Oh the loo, I've heard terrible things about kids drowning in the loo.'

'We'll get lots of locks for everything.'

'Maybe we could just raise the loo. Put it on a dais or something.'

We get quotes from a builder, plumber and electrician. The combined cost, including labour and parts, of having every window, plug socket and the bath, loo and basin raised higher would come to about thirty-three grand. So I've decided it might be cheaper to relax about all the hazards.

To be honest, I have always found it naff walking into the houses of friends who have kids, and having to circumnavigate my way around door- and window-locks, complex stair-gates, endless mesh protectors, fireguards and softening devices on low, sharp corners. But now that I'm pregnant I intend to turn our flat into Kiddy Alcatraz – budget allowing, of course. Bleach and sharp knives only reachable once you've got past the lasers and alarm system.

I seek solace during yet another stress- and worry-filled day watching *Bergerac* on UK Gold. I find John Nettles' cornflower-blue eyes strangely comforting.

145 days to go ...

AN UNMEMORABLE DAY'S FILMING. Some poor sap found some other poor sap and they were rewarded with a date from hell to a bowling alley.

I realised today that pregnancy has made me much more suspicious of people. A primitive reflex, perhaps, when you needed to defend your unborn from sabre-toothed moggies. I view everyone as a potential enemy or threat through lizardy, half-closed eyes. This morning Henrietta was sitting quite near my handbag and I had the strange impulse that she was going to pinch something from it. Henrietta drives a Land Rover to work and her dad's something big in the City – what need could she possibly have for a bottle of Gaviscon, a purse with 60p in it or my library card? I feel like an Alsatian guard dog. Come near my baby, and I'll maul your hand off.

144 days to go ...

I HATE ROY.

Roy is employed by Duchess as an all-round security bod, someone to keep an eye on things generally and make sure that members of the public don't swipe any equipment while we're on location. He is a ruddy, portly type with a spitty, sibilant diction and a leer. Added to that he has a remarkable belief in his own jokes, which he'll repeat to anyone within spitting range. He also has a very annoying habit of greeting me every day with: 'Hello, Mum.' He delivers it with a slightly slimy sexual edge, and I find it unfathomably sinister. It's all part of that unspoken way you become everybody's property when you're pregnant. Like some awful cuddly mascot that everybody can pat.

And today I hated Roy more. I think my hormones have gone into overdrive. No sooner had I got into work, Roy collared me, his eyes swishing down over my breasts to take in the sight of my ever-bulging tum, and said, 'How's Mum today?' I had to take myself off to the Ladies – we were filming in a leisure centre in Loughborough – and literally cool myself down under a cold tap. Not only did he leer at me – but he used *the third sodding person*! That means I no longer exist! Everything about me has been erased. Every nuance of my persona, every detail of my character has been smeared out of existence by this odious man. I was in a foul mood all day and left the leisure centre by a back exit so that I wouldn't have to see Roy's greasy face.

143 days to go ...

THINGS DON'T GET ANY BETTER. I have the morning off and decide to use it fruitfully choosing paint for the nursery. I saunter into Harris Hardware around the corner and flick through the colour swatches. Then I feel his presence. It's Jim, one of the Harris employees – a short tubby man with large Reactalite glasses. He has that air of aggression which only the short man possesses, as if he might suddenly jump out of his stonewash denim jacket and clock you round the head with a pre-cut length of pine. I try to ignore him, and concentrate on refining my colour scheme ideas.

'Haven't seen you on the telly for a while.'

'No, we've been doing other things.'

'What, opening fêtes and that?'

I feel my hormones rising. Keep your cool, Mel. Think of meadows, think of John Nettles, think of the baby. I can feel Jim's breath somewhere near my shoulder. I turn to face him. He looks down at my bump, laughs and calls over to the other lads in the shop.

'Look at this! Are you expecting twins or what?'

That's it. The hormones have flown straight to the place behind my eyes and I push a finger into Jim's stone-washed front.

'I'm a prima gravida expectant mother, Jim, in my second trimester. I have one baby inside my uterus and I'd appreciate it if you didn't make pathetic jokes about it, all right?'

'Wooooh!' he squeaks. 'Keep your knickers on, love. I thought you were supposed to be a comedian.'

'There is nothing funny about having a baby, Jim. It's bloody hard work, you feel bloody tired all the time ...' I can feel the tears welling up '... and you're a prat!'

I burst into tears and throw the colour swatches into Jim's face. All

I can think about as I run down the street is my naff choice of insult.

As I tell Dan about ghastly Jim when I get home, gasping the story out through tears, the whole Roy story comes out too, and I throw in a horrible neighbour called Neil, who made some quip to me about 'being in the pudding club', for good measure.

Dan is a model of understanding. He says I've developed an extreme hormonal reaction to men with one-syllable names. He's probably next.

142 days to go ...

My first block of filming is now out of the way. Lucinda McCleod showed up on the last day and managed a sinister stretched smile. She glanced at my bump, said 'I prefer dogs to children' and was gone.

Have been on the phone solidly today. Caught up with Mum who told me that if I started to suffer from heartburn I should watch out because it could mean that the baby will be very flatulent. Tried to speak to various mates to keep them up to speed with the pregnancy – weirdly got a lot of answerphones. I even managed to get hold of my elusive friend Pen.

Pen does A&R for a record company and is always being flown out to exotic places to discover new acts. She's got two tickets to see Marilyn Manson in two weeks and wonders if I'd like to go.

'Yeah, brilliant!' I reply immediately. 'I'd love to see her.'

'Marilyn Manson's a man, Mel.'

'Whatever. I just want to get out of the house!'

141 days to go ...

THE PHONE GOES AT FOUR O'CLOCK in the morning. My immediate reaction is to pull on my palazzo pants. It must be a filming day. Oh God, where are we going today? Manchester? Grimsby? Dan takes the call.

'It's Amanda.'

'What?' I pull the phone over to my side of the bed. 'Amanda! Are you OK?'

I barely recognise the small, snuffly voice.

'Look, I need your help. I've gone into labour. And it's London Fashion Week.'

'Is that strictly relevant? Am I missing something?'

'Tash was supposed to be my birth partner but she's doing PR for it.'

'And where's Roger?'

'Dubai.'

Brilliant. Roger the cipher-husband fails to be present yet again. I'm amazed he didn't appear on a satellite link-up at his own wedding. I try now to do my best calm, slightly patronising voice, the one I use when giving foreign tourists directions.

'OK. Now. Are you breathing?'

'Of course I'm breathing, otherwise I'd be dead.'

Ignore this. Women in labour tend to be irrational.

'How often are the ... the ... you know ...'

Dan chips in lazily from his side of the bed, 'Contractions.'

'Yes, contractions, thanks, Dan.'

'Oh God, I don't know, every few minutes, I think.'

'Right. And do you think you've started ... you know ... the cervix?'

'Dilating.' That's Dan again. Thank goodness one of us is reading the sensible lady doctor's book.

'I've no idea. How the hell can I see up there?'

'OK, and what about your waters?'

But all I can hear at this point is a sort of whoop of pain from Amanda.

'There's ... another ... one ... ohmyGod that's painful ... mmm ... can you ... come ... over?'

'Me?'

'I'm sorry, Mel, but you're just the only person I could think of.'

A classic Amanda backhanded compliment, like a sock in the guts.

'I'll call a cab. I'll be with you in half an hour. Stay right where you are, and try to get comfy ... er ...'

Dan's sitting up now, fully alert.

'Tell her to run a warm bath and try to ride the contractions with her breathing. Not little fussy shallow breaths, but good, deep, nasal inhalations. Tell her that adopting the doggy position can help to ease back pain.'

He's unnerving me now. I hang up, disturbed by the idea of Dan thinking about Amanda in the doggy position.

'Why on earth is she calling me? She's got loads of friends.'

'But they're not muckers,' says Dan.

'I'm hardly Amanda's mucker!'

'But you have known her for a long time.'

A terrible thought strikes me.

'Oh God, I'll probably see her bits.'

'Yes, you will undoubtedly see her bits. And a lot more besides.'

'I haven't seen her bits since we were in my paddling pool.'

'Look, are you sure you should go? I don't want you getting too stressed.'

'Well, it sounds distinctly like there's no one else there for her. I've got to go.'

The cab arrives and Dan bundles me in. As I pull away, Dan jogs beside the cab, holding on to the window.

'Tell her to try to avoid episiotomy – and ask the midwife for hot pads on the perineum!'

Dan's little lecture is swiftly curtailed as the cab gains sudden speed. I look back and catch sight on him, standing in his pyjamas in the middle of the road.

Considering she's in quite a lot of pain and, I presume, a fairly advanced stage of labour, Amanda looks pretty good as she opens the door in freshly laundered yoga slacks, a spotless T-shirt and a spray of something Calvin Kleiny around her neck and hair.

A neat collection of Louis Vuitton luggage, including two tiny cases for the baby, waits by the door.

'Do you want a cup of tea, Amanda? Do you want to sit down?'

'No I'm better just … pacing … Mmmm … I think another one's coming … oh God, they're more frequent … yes … Wooooh! Here it comes.'

Amanda makes a noise rather like she would have done at Parsonage Mead on the sidelines of a netball match. It's disturbing.

'Have you phoned for an ambulance?'

'It's on its way.'

'OK.'

'And listen. Thanks so much for coming. Bloody Tash. And Emma has been a total nightmare too. I tried to phone her but she was on the dancefloor at China White's and she couldn't even hear me.'

We arrive in one piece at one of London's most exclusive postcodes. I am expecting the usual TV hospital drama scenario – a whole load of stressed-out men and women in green pyjamas, who rush you on to a trolley and stick a drip in your arm. But not here at Amanda's chosen private maternity unit. It feels rather like arriving at a premiere. A smart uniformed man levers us out of the car, someone else arrives to take the luggage, and we're guided through some swishing smoked-glass doors into what looks like a smart hotel lobby. The sort where you get Bulgari jewellery and headscarves for sale behind a glass case.

'Mrs Smythe? We've been expecting you. And is this lady also in for delivery?'

'I'm only six months pregnant,' I say dourly.

'I'm so sorry. Can I take madam's name?'

'She's Mel.'

'A relative?'

'My best friend,' says Amanda.

We really are not best friends, but this is no time for a schoolgirl huff. I bite my lip. Amanda is whisked off in a wheelchair down a corridor which has the comforting sounds of Clannad piping through it. She cranes her head into every room that we pass to see if she can spot any celebrities. I sort of jog behind.

We are shown into the Nightingale Suite, a large carpeted set of rooms with all the creature comforts. It just about succeeds in masking the slightly menacing air of the medical that loiters just out of sight. There's a large monitoring thing on wheels placed discreetly behind an elegant curtain and a metal stool lurking underneath the crisp valance of the bedspread.

'Amanda, you get your own fruit basket! How cool is that?'

The luggage man looks disdainfully at me, before bowing out of the room.

'He was wearing a bow-tie! A bow-tie in a hospital. Wait till I tell Dan.'

There is a low divan for partners to recline on, to one side of the main maternal throne, and on a nest of tables beside it every magazine known to woman – fantastic! I throw myself on to it with real joy.

'*Heat*, *Hello!* and *OK*, please,' says Amanda immediately. I rather pompously pick up *Country Life* and we spend a nice few minutes absorbed in our respective reading matter.

There is a knock at the door and a minion enters with full menu as well as a wine list. The only thing you'd get in an NHS establishment would be a whine list: 'My bed's uncomfortable'; 'Can you tell that woman to get her kids out of this ward'; 'I want pethidine'.

Our next visitor is a suave South African in his late forties. By the look of him I'd say his favourite location is the tennis court. He has the affable, relaxed air of the very tanned and the very rich.

'I'm Mr de Vaal. I'm your consultant and I hope your stay with us will be very pleasant. Please call me if you experience any difficulties.' He winks at both of us and checks his clipboard. 'And are we opting for a Caesar today?'

For one minute I think he's referring to a salad on the menu.

'No, Mr de Vaal. I'm going to go natural if I can.'

'No scarring, hey? You want to wear that bikini at St Tropez next summer!'

More winking. What a creep.

I sense Amanda needs a bit of space, so I decide to get out of Nightingale for ten minutes and explore.

It's the strangest hospital I've ever been into. Unnervingly quiet. The lights have been lowered as if it's a dinner party. There are no wards, no raucous nurses' laughter, or big industrial mops prowling the corridors, no children screeching or psychotic out-patients complaining. Everything is hushed and dimmed. And the spookiest thing is you can't hear a single baby in this place. They must be somewhere. Perhaps they're hidden away, behind thick, sound-proofed walls.

I wander down several corridors past a couple of Eurotrashy dads checking their Rolex watches, talking into mobile phones, and an enormous gang of veiled Saudi women. On the way back I stop at the coffee machine. As I wait for my cinnamon cappuccino, I see a very familiar-looking man in sunglasses, shambling towards me jingling some change. Is it? Oh my God, it is! I've gone scarlet and I haven't even looked round yet. I keep my gaze fixed on the coffee machine. I'm so excited my right knee's trembling. He and his brother invented Brit Pop – I've got all of their albums and even had a haircut like them in the late eighties!

I try to look nonchalant and start to hum lightly. It helps me keep my equilibrium until I realise that I'm actually humming one of his most famous songs. With quick yet subtle modulation I turn the song into 'Got To Pick a Pocket or Two' from the musical *Oliver*. I think I get away with it.

I'm not going to let this opportunity slip away. Sue told me that she once saw him in the street and he nodded to her and said, 'All right, kid?' albeit quite gruffly. That's a good start, he obviously knows who we are. I turn to him with my most cheeky of smiles and am met with the blank, slack-jawed face of Cool Britannia.

'Cinnamon!' I say cheerily. 'What will they think of next?'

He says nothing, just sniffs and rattles his change.

'So what are you doing here?' I say as an ice-breaker.

''Avin' a baby,' he replies, without even looking at me.

'Me too. I mean, not actually me but a friend of mine, I mean I'm due to have a baby quite soon but I'm just here with her because her birthing partner couldn't make it.'

Silence. He selects his coffee. Black. No sugar. Of course.

'I think you met my friend once. Sue? Apparently you said "All right, kid" to her.'

Now I'm afraid I make a very bad error here. When saying the words 'All right, kid', I actually attempt a little impression of him – *to his face*. His reaction is to take his coffee out of the dispenser. Now of course what I should do here is wrap it all up and head back to the Nightingale Suite to repair the tatters of my pride. But no. Like some death-wish victim I blunder on into the minefield.

'Sue? Sue Perkins? We're presenters, Mel and Sue. We used to do a lunchtime programme.'

He starts to chew his cheek. 'Never watch that crap. I don't get up till three.'

And with that he turns on his be-plimsolled heels and wanders off down the corridor. I try to catch my breath but I am winded with shame.

Things seem to have progressed in Nightingale while I've been committing social suicide. A midwife and her team have moved Amanda into her adjoining bathroom, and are helping her into what looks like an enormous Jacuzzi. She is starting to make quite a lot of noise at this point. It's still the kind of stiff-upper-lip Prizegiving Day cheer with added moan on the end.

'Sorry, I just went to get a coffee.'

'Right, well, you can make yourself useful. Stand up at Mum's top end, will you, and be supportive.'

Amanda is starting to pant a bit and declares rather gamely that she needs to do a poo.

'That's good, Amanda. That's good,' says the midwife encouragingly.

'Should I fetch some lavatory paper?' I suggest.

I'm told, in terms that make it clear they think I'm about as useful as a small child, that this is a sign the baby's head is coming down the birth canal. Dan would have known that. The midwife looks Amanda directly in the eye, like a boxing coach. 'Listen. We're going to get this baby out. When you feel another contraction I want you to start the pushing. Chin down into your chest, a really strong, deep push. Not just growling in your throat, that'll just give you a sore throat. I want real pushing. OK, my love?'

This woman is good. She is totally in control and we all know it. Amanda nods, moans and looks like she might be ready to die. I suddenly feel that I don't want to be here. I'm not sure that I'm going to be able to take this. But Don King barks at me again.

'Stroke Mum's hair out of her eyes.'

It feels weird to be stroking Amanda's head. I think this is the first physical contact I've had with her since playing Hide the Custard Cream when we were youngsters. Oh God. This is it. This is the moment.

'You're doing great, Amanda. Really great. Keep going.' I lightly stroke her wet hair.

She smiles weakly and starts panting in earnest. 'God … too … painful …' Then she lets out what I can only describe as something bovine. A cross between a bellow and a very intense mooing. I have to suppress the desire to laugh. The midwives move into action and urge her to push, push, feel the zenith of the contraction and then really push like mad.

'Come on! Nearly there! Nearly there!'

The same routine carries on for what seems like hours – in reality it's no more than twenty minutes.

'I can see the head!' announces one of the midwives.

'Bloody … Roger,' shouts Amanda. 'What … a … bloody … bastard.'

'Too right!' I agree rather too loudly.

At which moment she lets out an elephantine roar and out of her little body slips an amphibious creature into the water. The colour of the water has turned to red and there are one or two floaters bobbing around. A midwife tactfully deals with these using a special little sieve.

'Good girl, Amanda! Good girl! You're nearly done!'

The midwives now act like a crack team of delicatessen workers.

They are snipping, tucking, weighing, slapping and cleaning. Amanda still has to push the placenta out, but the worst is over for her. She lies her head back on the side of the bath and wallows in glorious relief. I am in floods.

'It's a boy!' I squeal.

A boy, a lovely miraculous boy that has just sprung into the world as it was always destined to. It's a squawking, wrinkled, waxy, plug-ugly mess of a boy, but it is the most beautiful thing that I've ever seen, and I'm not even his mother.

'Oh God, he looks just like Roger!' is Amanda's only comment at this juncture, but as she takes him in her arms, her eyes fill with tears, and she starts whispering rubbish into his little ear. I sincerely hope that he soon learns to filter out 90 per cent of this rubbish, which will bombard him over the next fifty or so years.

Mini-Roger cries lustily, and Amanda announces that in an hour, after bonding with her baby, she'd like a large dose of Temazepam and could one of the midwives possibly take care of him? I've had mixed feelings for Amanda over the years, but at this point in time I feel nothing but wholehearted respect for the woman.

I'm regaling Dan with all of the gory details on the phone, when I see the popstar and his tottering wife, in shades and stilettos, leave the hospital. As the smoked-glass doors swish open, there is a blaze of paparazzi flashbulbs. He turns his usual V sign into a V for Victory. The paps go wild. Their daughter has been displayed to the world, ready for a life of tabloid pages and strange, celebrity-infested events.

Meanwhile, back in Nightingale, Amanda is enjoying a blissful tranquillised sleep while a minion prepares vases for the inevitable onslaught of bouquets. Roger is on his way back from Dubai – nice that he can make it – and a variety of people including her yoga teacher and mother are pencilled in for an audience the following morning. I'm missing my bed and my Dan. I feel absolutely shattered, but I can't resist hunkering down next to the sleeping form of mini-Roger, him in his cot, me on the divan. I dream of the popstar in a farmyard, on all fours and bellowing one of his hits.

140 days to go ...

I RECEIVE A MESSAGE from Amanda telling me that, according to her consultant Mr de Vaal, she had a textbook birth. Textbook pregnancy, textbook birth, apparently even Roger showed up in a textbook-type way with armfuls of presents. No sign of any textbook gratitude for me though, her so-called best friend. I don't even warrant a thank you. I could quite happily never see her shallow Parsnips Weed face again.

Dan points out gently that I seem to be a bit moody at the moment and I bite his head off. But the truth is, he's right – I'm turning into a sourpuss. The thing that's getting on my wick is this: I have entered the period of time that is supposed to see me oozing fertile gorgeousness from every pore and radiating a glowing sense of mellow well-being, my so-called blooming period. Instead, I'm blooming hideous, cantankerous and grumpy.

I've been sold a lie. In the TV lady doctor's book there are pictures of women in this second trimester wafting around with supermodel skin and muted autumnal clothes, collecting herbs from the garden or walking along a beach with their life partner, laughing as they try to avoid the waves from splashing their pristine deck shoes. Or there's mum-to-be at home, smiling serenely at her computer while a pair of glasses on chains rest lightly on her accountancy work. All right, I know they've got to try to sell pregnancy as life-affirming and wonderful, but this is fantasy. Where are *we*? Where are the pictures of us women with spotty jowls and blown-up Sumo wrestler bodies? Where are the action shots of us puffing and panting as we bend over to winch our knickers up over our girths? Where are the close-ups of our puffy faces which have lost all humour and zest, and which now sit dribbling in front of repeat episodes of *Shoestring*? I am perfectly ready to accept that certain women just look fabulous when they're pregnant, but I do not want to see their silly smiley faces paraded before me.

It is also the case that friends cannot remain in a state of ecstatic excitement for the full nine months of your pregnancy. They do have their own lives to lead. I sat with a mate in the pub the other night who was pretty distraught about his love life.

'She just doesn't understand me any more, Mel.'

'Mmm. I know the feeling. My midwife's a bit like that with me. I mean I told her that I'm rhesus negative and that I need an injection of anti d at my thirtieth week, and she just forgot to put it into my notes.'

'I think we might be splitting up.'

'Mmm. Did you know that having a baby is the major cause of people splitting up? It's just so stressful and such a big deal that a lot of couples' relationships just buckle under it.'

'She keeps flirting with this guy at work just to torment me – you know the routine, batting the eyelashes, showing him the cleavage.'

'Mmm. Oh my God that reminds me! Have you ever seen the *disgusting* range of breast-feeding shirts you can buy? I've got this catalogue and there's a rugby shirt with a flap that does up with poppers that you can pull down for easy breast-feeding access. A rugby shirt! How grim is that?'

The poor guy lasted about twenty minutes before fleeing from the pub. And fair enough. I have become a bore. I simply must keep myself in check.

134 days to go ...

FINALLY GOT THE CHANCE to talk to Pawel.

We sit down at the kitchen table and I embark on the usual monologue, filling in the gaps where he would normally speak. I talked about what he must be doing at the moment, how his PhD must be going, how he must be filling his free time. He smiles occasionally and twitches his moustache, which I notice actually has dandruff in it.

'Now, Pawel, you may have noticed *this!*' I say, pointing to my stomach.

Pawel laughs. I laugh too.

'Like Polish army officer,' says Pawel, and chuckles so much that his moustache quivers.

'Er ... sorry?'

'Army very lazy. Much food!' He laughs a whole lot more.

My smile drops. 'No, Pawel. I'm pregnant.'

He looks blank.

'I'm having a baby, Pawel!' I do the international mime for 'baby', which involves the rocking of arms.

'Ah yes! Baby! Very nice! Very good!' And he shakes my hand vigorously as if we've just signed a treaty.

Now for the tricky bit.

'So, Pawel. There will be a few changes in the house. You know, when the baby arrives.'

He says nothing and stares at me. I crash on.

'So, you might want to, you know, think about moving? Another flat? Very noisy here with baby!'

Well done, me. Eviction order signed, sealed, delivered. The penny (or in Pawel's case, zloty) finally drops. He grins in recognition.

'Ah yes, no worry, Mel! I like noise of baby. I can stay in room. No problem, baby reminds me of Poland.'

I can't face this.

129 days to go ...

THE *EX MANIAC* FILMING has finished and the obligatory enormous bouquet arrived on cue yesterday. The usual note accompanied it: 'Darling Mel, Duchess loves you! You're a star. XXXXX.' It is completely unmerited. They should be sending flowers to the ordinary Joe Public suckers who will be slaughtered on screen to get the cheap laughs that make the programme tick.

My mood hasn't shifted. It lingers like a stifling fog over me, the flat, and poor Dan. In a desperate attempt to lift my spirits I opt for that tried and tested girly stand-by: a trip to the hair salon for a me-time makeover, some general pampering and the universal balm of vacuous gossip. I book it for tomorrow.

To brighten up the daily raft of junk mail and bills, Dan and I received today an invitation to a party: 'Please come to the Naming Ceremony of Doric Sage Jimi O'Brien.' Little Doric is the son of an extremely earthy friend of my sister from her CND days. Jools seems to have latched on to me with sinister enthusiasm, far in excess of our standing relationship, since she's heard about my mother-to-be status.

And quite a set of names they have chosen too. Doric? A little too close to 'dork' for my liking. Perhaps they have a career mapped out for him as a columnist. Sage? Now that will definitely ensure he gets the stuffing knocked out of him once he gets to school. And Jimi, for goodness' sake? I'm presuming after Hendrix – a transparently vain attempt by his parents to look rebellious and cool. We must come up with some names ourselves before we are forced by last-minute angst to opt for something we'll regret.

128 days to go ...

'SO WHEN'S IT DUE?' asks Melissa, my designated shampooer and rinser.

'December.'

'That's nice. Boy or girl?'

'We don't know. Want to keep it a surprise.'

'That's nice. Is it your first?'

'Yes.'

'That's nice.'

It's lovely that people are immediately so interested in one's special condition. You can get stuck into a really interesting chat about yourself straight away, and in a hairdressing situation it also diverts the conversation away from imminent holiday plans.

'So, going away anywhere then?'

Then again.

'Er ... I don't know. Possibly a weekend in Suffolk – Aldeburgh maybe, or Dunwich.'

A pause.

'That's nice,' Melissa says unconvincingly.

I have been to this particular hairdresser before – I was sent here by Duchess Productions to be spruced up for the job. It is rather too flash for my tastes but I'm too lazy to find anywhere else. The stylists dress in black lycra and rollnecks like one of those dance troupes that you used to see on Saturday night light entertainment shows – *The Brian Rogers Connection* springs to mind. They swish around in vague unison with their smooth black contours and pert bottoms, and big clips sticking in their waistbands. Mine is a senior stylist and her name is Suzanne.

'So, what are we doing for you today, Mel?'

'I need to be lifted. Something radical. Goodbye old me, hello new.'

I can tell Suzanne's impressed.

'Groovy! And good to do something to complement the way you're looking now.'

Which is a polite way of saying that I look like a middle-aged librarian. She hands me a file with weird loops of hair in them.

'Colour. I think something really strong but warm would be nice. And we should go bold with the style. Let's chop away all this deadwood round here.' She handles the mess of hair like a fishmonger with a slimy guppy. 'How about something fun like a New Millennium Bowl?'

'Wow! What's that?'

I'm liking the sound of this a lot. Her use of the word 'bold' thrills me. 'Bowl' is slightly worrying, but I'm keeping an open mind.

'It's such a cute look.' She hands me another file full of gamine faces with bowl haircuts. I have to say, they look just like bowl haircuts of old to me.

'Aren't they fab?' says Suzanne. 'They've got a kind of ironic *Space 1999* vibe about them.'

'Yes, they do!' I lie, but I'm starting to haver. 'Maybe something along these lines, but not quite so bowly, Suzanne? I'm not sure my face can carry it off.'

'With your face the bowl would look gorgeous, Mel. Tell you what, let's make a start and see how we get on?'

'Yeah! Actually, I'm going to a Marilyn Manson gig tomorrow – I need something bold!'

'Marilyn Manson? Cool!' Suzanne is bowled over.

That does it. One New Millennium Bowl sold to the pregnant lady in the dungarees!

Three hours later I leave the salon feeling hot, flustered, itchy and still damp around the neck. It's all very well looking at yourself in the salon mirror for a final appraisal, but you can really only judge a new haircut in a neutral environment.

I go into a clothes shop and the assistant's eyes instantly flicker to my hair. A secluded mirror confirms my fears. I have been given a bloody bowl haircut. It's not New Millennium, it's not even *Space 1999* – this is Lincolnshire 1399. I look like a medieval peasant. It is starkly, uncompromisingly cut, emphasising my ever-weakening jowls and rather patchy complexion. Oh, and the colour is heinous – a deep matt chocolate brown. It looks like an NHS wig. Quick, get some lipstick on, that always helps. A sweep of pink pastel over the lips – no, that's worse. I look like one of my old school dinner ladies. I'm close to tears and mumbling to myself. No amount of ruffling it with spittle can shift the immovable, cement-like bowl. This is a disaster.

Never ever have a radical haircut when you're pregnant. Just trust me on this.

'It's not actually that bad,' says Dan, gingerly stroking the bowl.

'Mmmrgggh Valerie Singleton mmmrgh.'

'I can't hear you with your face in the pillow.'

I have been lying on our bed like this for the last three hours. I will never ever leave the house again.

'It'll grow pretty quickly, and anyway, I think you look ... nice.'

'I don't want NICE! And no one looks NICE at gigs!' I wail.

'You could always wear a hat tomorrow. What about that one you wore last summer?' he suggests.

'That's a wedding hat, Dan. I cannot go to see Marilyn Manson at the Brixton Academy in a wedding hat.'

'Well, what about the Indian one – that's cool.'

'I wore that on my year off. I'll look like Milly Tant out of *Viz*.'

'Look. You should be able to wear exactly what you want. That's what Manson's supposed to be about, isn't he? Freedom of expression? Standing out from the crowd? Come on, don't be a wimp, it's only a haircut, for God's sake,' and with that he rather impressively sweeps out of the room. Damn it, he's right.

127 days to go ...

I HAVE OPTED VERY MUCH FOR Dan's freedom-of-expression look this evening. I am in denim dungarees – I just couldn't face taking them off, they are becoming my second skin – a velveteen tracksuit top, a pair of gym shoes and my little Indian hat, which has got bits of beading and mirror all around the edge. The chocolate bowl is visible but only in fringe form, broken up with gel to form chunks across my forehead. I have put on quite a bit of fake tan to compensate for the pasty face, which gives me a satsuma-like hue, but the lighting on the tube's always harsh and it will be dark at the gig. I would describe this evening's look as 'brave'.

It is only when I approach the Brixton Academy that I realise just quite how brave. The people swarming around are straight out of an urban post-Apocalyptic circus, all leather and bizarre piercings. There are perforated chins, eyelids and even hands. One boy can hardly move his mouth he's got so many tin-tacks in it. Every time he talks to his girlfriend his studs go clickety-click. He's not sterilising those every night with cotton wool and witch hazel. And I wouldn't want to be either of them in a freak lightning strike – they'd go up like a crisp.

Now don't get me wrong, I dabbled with the goth movement myself when I was fourteen. But that was just a bit of purple eyeliner and back-combed sugared hair of a Saturday night. Right now, amid the bum-length hair extensions and weird white contact lenses, I have never in my life felt so out of place. Actually I tell a lie. I once wore traditional Polish costume to a fancy dress party where everyone else went as Adam Ant.

I scan the crowd for Pen. I need to find a friendly face. After fifteen minutes of battling my way through hair and pierced flesh, I hear a familiar voice.

'Mel? Mel!'

I turn round. Before me is a vision in fishnets, sculpted hair, trapeze-artiste's breeches and top-hat. It is all jet-black and finished with a Victorian high-neck, ruffled shirt, which is totally diaphanous. Everything is visible.

'Pen?'

She gives me an ecstatic hug. Her pupils are warmly dilated. She introduces me to a guy in a black tutu.

'This is Marco.'

'Ah! The Black Swan!'

No reaction. Marco gives me a discreet once-over and then immediately looks away. He is clearly mortified to be seen with me.

'What's with the Greenham Common look, Mel?' says Pen, and then cackles with laughter. I laugh too.

'You should have told me it'd be like this,' I wail, 'then I could have worn something a bit groovier!'

'What, your "Women Are Angry" T-shirt?' More laughter.

God, it's good to see her, she's like an injection of pure caffeine to the system.

'How are you feeling, darling?' She lights up a cigarette.

'Yeah, pretty good. My midwife says that the baby's doing just fine. And I don't feel sick any more which is just such a rel—'

'Drink?' Pen interjects hastily.

Thank goodness for that. I was on the brink of rolling out the current dimensions of the foetus. We squash against the bar.

'Double JD with Coke,' shouts Marco to the barman. 'Pen?'

'Double vodka and tonic.'

'Mel?'

'Half a lime and soda please, Marco. No ice!'

Pen and I bag a table, and I turn to her confidentially.

'I never trust ice in these places, the water might be infected and I just can't risk getting food poisoning at the moment.'

Pen stifles the tiniest of yawns and her eyes water ever so slightly.

'So. Marco. Is he your latest man?'

'Nah, he's more of a fuck buddy really.'

If I'd had my lime and soda I'd have choked on it right there.

'Your what?'

'When I want a shag I just call him up and vice versa.'

'Cool,' I say, trying to sound at ease with the idea.

'I'm single at the moment,' Pen tells me. 'I was seeing this married woman. Nightmare. Never get involved with anyone straight, that's my motto.'

'Oh God, yeah.'

'How's Dan?'

'He's brilliant. And straight.'

Pen laughs.

'Pen, I've had a terrible haircut.'

'I know, love. I can see. It's a bowl, isn't it?'

Pen starts to laugh, and so do I. I can't stop. I laugh so much I nearly wet myself.

The vibe inside the auditorium is electric. Thankfully we've got seats, although everyone is up on their feet. Manson looks like the Child-catcher from *Chitty Chitty Bang Bang*. He is amazing. Everyone has their arms up, hands in the shape of horns, and Pen and Marco are jumping around like dervishes. She looks fabulous. She'll drink and smoke herself into oblivion tonight and then tip up at work, dishevelled but still beautiful, with a glint in her eye and some new stories with which to shock her colleagues. She takes life for everything it's got. All I, on the other hand, demand from life at the moment are big bras and hot milky drinks. And the only drama in my life at the moment is *The Archers* omnibus.

My limbs are suddenly heavy and the music's starting to crush my head. I sit down. As the gig goes on, my buttocks begin to feel like squashed blood oranges, and I shift from one to the other to keep the circulation going. The girl members of Manson's troupe are now naked bar some jackboots, and are goose-stepping around the stage. The audience are lapping it up, the place is throbbing. But I need to get out of here. I need to breathe some fresh air. I need to take this itchy hot hat off. I need to lie down. I tap Pen's shoulder and point to the exit. She doesn't care. She puts her thumbs up and then turns back to Manson.

I'm the only one leaving early and the bouncers give me a patronising look as they open the doors for me. There's a cab and I collapse into the back, head still pulsating. I'm relieved to be out. Yet I'm envious of Pen's verve, of her freedom. I feel sad because all that's over for me. I'm going to be a mummy. That's what's happening. I'm being slowly mummified. The bandages are getting ever closer, and will soon be bound tightly around me. I'll be locked in a tomb, sealed away for a hundred years, only to be released for Sports Day or PTA meetings.

The poor cab driver. He kindly supplies me with some mansize tissues, as I gently blubber all the way home.

'Cheer up, love, it might never happen.'

126 days to go ...

I WAKE UP TO FIND the pillow streaked with chocolate brown hair dye. I start crying again immediately. Dan has mastered the uncanny skill of being able to offer me his shoulder to cry on while he's still sleeping. As he drifts into consciousness I tell him of my mummification fears. He thinks about it.

'Well, how do you think I feel?'

I'm ashamed to say that I haven't really given this question much thought.

'Well, pretty OK, aren't you?'

Dan looks at me. 'I feel a bit weird sometimes ... Down, I suppose. I see all those knackered-looking dads in the supermarket, desperately clinging on to the vestiges of their hair, still wearing trendy jeans and trainers in an effort to stay young, and it makes me feel depressed. I feel a bit useless too. At least you have something tangible inside of you. I feel like a bit of a twat on the sidelines.'

All these months I have been swimming in Lake Me, I never even realised Dan felt remotely worried about anything.

'And then I think about how lucky we are. I saw Rob the other day – you know he and his wife have been having IVF for the past year? He says it's terrible. It's painful, expensive and stressful, and it might not even work. Imagine that? If we couldn't have kids? I know the baby's going to turn everything upside down, but you know what? I don't mind. We'll be fine. We'll still be the same essentially. Just poorer and more tired. So what?'

I lie in Dan's arms without saying anything for twenty minutes. I feel better for the first time in weeks.

120 days to go ...

A WEEK LATER I'm lying on the sofa watching a really terrible weepy Channel 5 film at three in the afternoon. My hand alternates between dipping into a big bag of Maltesers and hovering over a six-pack of M&S Scotch eggs. The Scotch egg is my new vice. Cheddar is *so* three months ago. As the Scotch egg and chocs meet and fizz away in enzyme hell somewhere in my guts, they cause little flutters in my tummy. Wow, quite a big flutter for one moment there. Then it strikes home – that isn't a Scotch egg! It's the baby!

It is. It's a little arm or leg, maybe even the head, butting against the side of its weird spongy cage. It's really there! It feels really nice actually, like when your eye ticks when you're tired, but in your tummy and quite a bit stronger.

When I was an au pair in Italy, I worked for a woman who used to talk to her bump through a plastic shower attachment, the old type that you hook on to the taps. We've got one of those, so I de-nozzle it from the bath and start with just a few simple introductions.

'Hello, my darling. This is your mother speaking. How are you in there? Hope you're enjoying the Scotch eggs!'

It feels good. It's important for the mothership to make contact with her little alien.

115 days to go ...

TODAY IS DORIC SAGE JIMI O'BRIEN'S BIG DAY and we are there to share it with him and his parents, Jools and Henry.

They live in a square in the East End of London that is still home to a few squatters. Jools and Henry secretly wish that they lived in a squat too, but Jools's trust fund has put paid to that. Still, they have tried to make the front of their house look as much like a squat as possible – radical slogans like 'Kenneth Baker, Education's Undertaker' are still visible, which Henry daubed on to the wall for the 1989 Grants not Loans march. Jools has transformed one of her flowerbeds into a mini Angolan minefield, complete with a little model of a boy with his foot blown off.

We ring on the 'bell' (a collection of recycled aluminium cans on string) and are greeted by the ever-jovial Henry, resplendent in a rainbow waistcoat and what look suspiciously like juggler's trousers. Big hugs all round and we are ushered straight into the back garden where the Naming Ceremony is about to commence.

We are a collection of around forty people, adults and kids. There are lots of sandals, braless breasts and quite a few berets too. Henry rings a little clay bell to get everyone's attention, and clears his throat.

'Guys. It's great that you're all here. I know some of you have come from afar, and Sandy, thanks for leaving the Terminal Five protesters at Heathrow to be with us today. That means an awful lot to us.'

Henry's speech is going well so far; he must have been in the Debating Society at Harrow.

'Jools and I conceived our beloved Doric,' oh no, his voice is cracking, 'in a tent at Avebury, in Wiltshire. We were pitched in a stone circle, and there was something magical about our lovemaking that night.'

Dan pinches my leg. Neither of us risk even glancing at each other for a second.

'Jools said that she knew my seed had been planted that night, and I dunno, we feel so, so blessed that it was. Doric is our be-all, our end-all and our forever-all.'

A smattering of applause at this. Henry's reeling them in. There are quite a few brimming eyes in the crowd.

'And I ask all of you now to come forward and join me and my own Gaia,' whereupon he smiles lovingly at Jools, 'as we charge our glasses with Toby's special mead – thanks for that, Tobes – and gather together around the rowan tree to name our darling fruit.'

I cannot help myself from letting out a loud snigger. The naming of a fruit? It reminds me of the Best Vegetable contest at the Leatherhead Harvest Festival.

At this point a woman in a kaftan strikes up on a fiddle and starts to half-sing, half-shout a song in honour of the baby.

'My emperor sits at my breast,' she warbles, 'my emperor sucks on my breast ...'

Dan is bruising my leg he's nudging it so hard. We all sort of huddle around poor little Doric, who must be getting alarmed at the amount of hessian closing in on him. Henry holds him up and shouts, 'Doric Sage Jimi! Be free, be unafraid, be you!'

And we all cheer and drink his health with Toby's mead, which I have to say tastes like manure.

Naming done with, we can get down to some serious buffet business, which has been laid out on a trestle underneath some trees. Just as I've stuffed my mouth with some cauliflower cutlet, Jools hugs me rather hard from behind and then shoves her beloved Doric into my arms while she hoiks her boob back into its jerkin. Doric looks a bit like Orson Welles, but of course I don't say so. He fixes me with his eye as if to say, 'So go on, then. Crack your boobs out, that's all I'm interested in.'

Jools's eyes momentarily fill with tears. 'Isn't he gorgeous?' she coos.

'Yes,' says Dan, a tad flatly.

'He's very ... imperial looking,' I add.

Jools looks worried. Imperial? Like a dictator? I've always thought that babies look like balding old tyrants from the history books:

Napoleon, Mussolini or Chairman Mao, and Jools' dobber of a son is no exception. Oh dear, some severe back-pedalling is required.

'I mean, he looks sort of knowing, and regal.'

'I think he looks like the Dalai Lama,' says Jools firmly.

'Yes, that's it,' I agree hastily, 'the Dalai Lama. Very Buddhist.'

Jools smiles. 'So how are you both doing? How's it going?' She pats my bump.

'Not too bad, Jools. It's due in December.'

'Oooh, lucky you! Sagittarius with Gemini rising! It'll be a real thinker.'

'That's great. I want it to think a lot,' says Dan, cussedly. I shoot him a look.

'So have you done your birth plan yet?' asks Jools.

'Birth plan? Er ... what's that exactly?'

'You write down exactly how you want your birth to go,' she says matter-of-factly. 'For example, I really wanted Henry to hold me from behind in the birthing pool,' I try not to think about this, 'and I absolutely didn't want any intervention unless strictly necessary. We were really lucky actually and I think the basil nosegay really helped.'

'I'm sorry?'

'It's a very popular white witch's method of pain relief. Strong sweet basil is formed into a little bundle and you attach it under your nose when you're contracting.'

Dan has turned to the buffet, his shoulders rising and falling.

'Oh right, I'll remember that, Jools.'

'What are you thinking in terms of pain relief?' she enquires gently.

'Pethidine, hopefully. They say it's like riding a rollercoaster.'

Jools's mouth has been left temporarily open by my revelation, giving Dan enough time to turn from the buffet and join us, his mouth stuffed with a canapé.

'Great pâté,' he mumbles.

'That's my placenta. I kept it and froze it. Isn't it lovely that we can all share in it?'

108 days to go ...

I'M OFF TO VISIT MY MUM for a couple of days. It'll be good to catch up with her. Dad will be way then, so she'll enjoy the company. And if we're going to be talking childbirth and babies then it's just as well that Dad's out of the way. He's fine with chat about Lithuanian horses giving birth, but any talk of ladies' bodily functions makes him queasy.

Dan sees me off at the station. Just before I board the train he pulls out *The Mothercraft Manual*, which, of course, I have failed to read.

'Your mum's bound to test you on it,' he says, then kisses me goodbye. 'Have a great time and relax.'

'And you're sure you don't mind dealing with Pawel?' I say with my most effective helpless, doe-eyed expression.

'Leave it to me.'

As the train pulls away and his tall frame recedes, I settle myself into the carriage. I do like a nice train journey. It's particularly gratifying at the moment as I'm getting lots of friendly smiles. At this stage of pregnancy, with the bump at last looking cheeky and clearly visible, people offer you an expression they'd normally reserve for the old family Labrador. If a passenger were to come up right here, roll me over and scratch my bulbous stomach, I wouldn't bat an eyelid.

As I get out my magazine, I feel a sudden hot flush – my hormones signalling a mild state of alert. I look up to see a body lumbering down the aisle towards me. It's a woman. And – how dare she! – she's pregnant. Everyone's giving her the family dog smile. I pray silently that she won't notice me and feel she has to join me at my table and compare notes.

She's just walking past when a silver-haired gent in the opposite seat leans forward and chuckles, 'I hope we're not going to have to prepare towels, hot water and soap for you ladies! Keep your legs crossed, eh?

We don't want any accidents!'

I smile politely. Crisis is averted, however, as she carries on down the aisle. I get out *The Mothercraft Manual* and hide behind it to forestall any more banter with Silver Fox.

I open the book at random and am greeted by the chapter 'The End of the Digestive Process', which deals with the appalling shock that 1950s Mum is going to face when confronted with her first faeces-infested nappy: 'There is nothing nasty about napkins.'

I titter audibly and ironically. But its old-fashioned quaintness soon turns ominous and my smile fades. This is post-war Britain where you must give birth with a stiff lower lip. On the birth itself it asks the question, 'Do you really want your husband to see you in such disarray?' I skip to the slightly less worrying post-natal pages and the rest of the journey passes in a blur of woollen bolero jackets, trifle recipes, welfare milk and starchy matrons with endless housewifely chores. As we roll into Leatherhead station and I close the book, I have one question: How on earth did anyone ever give birth in the Fifties? Thankfully I know a woman who has the answer.

107 days to go ...

'THOSE DUNGAREES ARE HIDEOUS! They're as bad as my elephant bags.'

'Elephant bags?' I say with a brittle edge to my voice. I think they're quite cool in a road protestor type of way.

'I made the most *dreadful* pair of trousers for myself when I was expecting. They were run up from grey flannel and viewed from behind your father said I looked exactly like an elephant. Some wag at church used to say to me, "Are you having twins, dearie?"'

My mind turns briefly to Jim in the hardware store.

Mum is pretty chuffed to see me and has made the last twenty-four hours a luxury experience. Whenever I sit down, a nest of tables magically unravels with tea and little homemade goodies on it. She has always made everything from scratch with ingredients I'd never dream of buying, like vanilla pods and gelatin. There's always a bowl of chicken stock in the fridge and she never has to weigh anything. For as long as I've been alive, there has continuously been some sort of casserole or stew on the go in the oven. When I attempt to cook I need a free ten hours with a long nap and a total change of clothes at the end of it. Mum just glides from dish to dish, humming 'Oh Ruddier Than the Cherry' as she goes.

She's sorted out a little pile of things for the baby and says there is more in the attic. There's a woollen vest with ribbon running through it and enormous woollen knickers to match, two pairs of little bootees and an all-in-one romper thing. All hand-knitted, of course.

'Mum, these are brilliant. Thank you so much!'

'They're from the Tiny Beau range of patterns. Handwash, I'm afraid, but you can always do them in your soaker buckets.'

I haven't got the heart to tell Mum that I fully intend to be using the disposable range of napkinwear. I've smelt that distinctive odour in my sister's house enough times to know the soaker bucket's simply not an option for me and Dan.

There is something about being back at home – possibly the central heating which is always turned up to greenhouse level – that makes me very yawny and want to go to bed early. We watch a Felicity Kendal drama with a box of chocolates and then Mum sends me to bed. She shoos me upstairs like she always used to, from behind, with a newspaper, but instead of scampering up them I kind of waddle like a constipated bear.

'I've set your Teasmade for eight, darling. Now get off to sleep quickly. You've got panda eyes.'

I hear her humming away as she gets ready for bed. For as long as I can remember Mum has been singing – sometimes quite loudly and in public. As a child I avoided going into shops with her whenever possible. Headscarf tightly tucked under her chin, her cherry lips would warble 'Pale Hands I Love' as she pondered a scrag end of beef in the butcher's. And when she came to pick me up from school, she couldn't just hang around the gates chatting like the other mums, she'd call to us from across the playground, waving wildly out of the Vauxhall Viva, 'Yoo-hoo! Melly! Katie! Yoo-hoo.'

I wanted to curl up in the corner of the playground like a little woodland animal and be taken away by the RSPCA. Nobody but nobody could embarrass me the way my mum could.

My friends were always surprised at how posh my mother sounded when they met her, because I used to affect the local Leatherhead mockney – a pre-punk suburban patois. Not quite Johnny Rotten; David Bowie possibly – a good Surrey boy himself. My classmates would ask me upfront why she sounded so different from me.

'I'm adopted,' I would mumble.

Michelle Hooper's mum wasn't embarrassing at all. I longed for a mum like Mrs Hooper. So cool with her shag perm, tight trousers and open-toed high sandals so that you could see her red nails. She looked like Olivia Newton-John in *Grease*. She wore an ankle chain and a chain round her waist in summer. She smelt of something nice and strong, and smoked and laughed a lot as she waited at the school gates. None of the other mums really talked to her. My mum once told me that she was 'NQOCD' (not quite our class dear), but Mrs Hooper didn't seem to care. She chatted up the school gardener and any other males that were around. My dad called her the Painted Lady, but I remember he was only too happy to assist her with the Guess the Weight of the Cake at the summer fête. She had a tinkly voice on account of her stage training, and she always picked Michelle up in her racy Cabriolet.

It was rumoured that the car had been given to her by Ed 'Stewpot' Stewart, the famed presenter of *Crackerjack*. The story went that he'd been Mrs Hooper's boyfriend for a while. Michelle had even been up to a television studio and seen the filming of *Crackerjack* and everything.

I longed to be Michelle Hooper. Her hair smelt deliciously of grease from the full breakfast her mum used to cook her every morning. We never had cooked breakfast. My mum thought it was vulgar. We had porridge and homemade brown bread.

While I'd been given a tracksuit for my tenth birthday, Michelle got a real Spanish dancer's dress for hers, complete with clackety shoes and shawl. How I loved that dress and longed to do the flamenco in it! Michelle used to have the best birthday parties. Mrs Hooper always laid on an entertainer of some sort. Once it was a woman who came and showed us all how to put on make-up – it was brilliant. We all went home happily looking like Child Beauty Pageant freaks. And everyone got their own going-home bag with a present. I got a plastic tiara one year. After one of my dos you were lucky to go home with a couple of conkers from one of our trees. Now, I'm not knocking conkers – we used to make little conker chairs and tables and sit our dollies on them – but given the choice I'd have the tiara any day.

Michelle was everything a little girl growing up in the seventies wanted to be. She was allowed to have very long hair, which was sometimes, oh lucky girl, done up in a bun. Mine was always cut into a pageboy for ease. She was always the first girl in the class to get things like the Sindy caravan (with working deckchairs), the pogo stick and Girls' World. I begged my mum to get me a Girls' World for Christmas. She refused on the grounds that she thought that it was sinister and, looking back on it, was probably right. Girls' World was basically a dismembered head that you could put make-up on, and there was a big dial in the back of its neck which, when rotated, released a mane of glorious bottle-blonde hair. Mum said if I wanted a Girls' World I could make my own, and presented me with an old football, a wig and a box of eye shadow.

Michelle left our school when she was eleven. Her mum landed a chorus part in a West End musical and they went off to the bright lights of London. I never knew what became of her. We still have a very faded photo of that tenth birthday party. Michelle looks glorious in the Spanish dress; the rest of us encircle her adoringly. I'm wearing a pair of dungarees and my hair has just been cut – by my mum, of course. As I drift off to sleep in a warm haze of childhood reverie, I'm jerked awake by the sudden, terrible realisation that I look exactly the same at thirty-three as I did when I was ten. I wriggle with shame and descend deep beneath my Holly Hobby duvet.

106 days to go ...

THE TEASMADE SPURTS and brrrings at exactly eight. Mum will have been up for hours, pottering and getting breakfast ready. This is the sort of house where the breakfast table is always laid the night before, rather like a well-run B&B. Just as you're finishing supper, your barely empty plate is replaced with a clean cereal bowl and side plate. Followed shortly by a whole raft of cereals and jams.

I head downstairs and join Mum in the kitchen. She is humming something familiar from the musical *Salad Days.*

'A piano, a piano!' She pronounces it 'piar-no'. 'We're looking for a piano!'

'Morning, Mum.'

'Still wearing that old dressing gown, I see. We'll have to get you something nice for the hospital or else they'll think you're a single mother!'

So far my visit has been incident-free and I'm not going to blow it all by arguing over the usual thorny issues. It'll only end in tears and I've shed enough of those this pregnancy to fill the Leatherhead Leisure Centre's pool several times over.

She has been busy. Laid out on newspaper in the living room is even more maternity stuff: an array of strange appliances, miniature furniture and dusty bags of odds and ends.

'Some more things for Baby. It's all very useful and I'm sure you can't afford to buy anything at the moment.'

'What do you mean?'

'Well, we haven't seen much of you on the box, dear, have we?'

'Mum, I've actually just finished a twenty-episode, neo-reality, daytime dating show.'

The old tones are beginning to creep back into my voice as if I were thirteen again.

'Don't talk like that, you sound like a hoyden.'

This is one of my mum's favourite words. She uses it for graffiti artists and people who walk up the down escalators in department stores.

'And it's daytime, dear. I'm sure it doesn't pay as well and nobody's going to see it anyway, are they?'

She has stepped way out of line here. I'm about to launch into my monologue on the commissioning policies of the various broadcasters when she starts to look sheepish.

'I'm sorry, dear, that came out the wrong way. And anyway, it's probably for the best. I mean you don't want to be on television when you're ... well ... looking ... you know ...'

Her voice peters out. My hackles are totally up now. I don't know exactly what hackles actually look like, but mine are fully erect, fluorescent orange and visible from Birmingham.

'When I'm looking what?'

'Well, dear, you're not quite as svelte as you were in your television days, are you?'

That's it. I make a snorting sound like a horse on a wintry day, and stalk out of the room. I may be thirty-three, but I can still flounce like a fourteen-year-old. I know the routine very well. Out of the kitchen and the lower lip starts to tremble somewhere around the bathroom landing. I clod upstairs with as heavy a tread as possible and then *whoof*! Stretch my length straight out on top of the bed. I'm sincerely hoping that the bed doesn't break.

I can't quite believe I'm doing this. That's the power of the mother. She can still reduce you to child-like status even if you're fast approaching middle age.

I leave it a decent half-hour before I emerge from my tragedy. I was sort of hoping that Mum would come up to my room and apologise, stroke my hair and tell me how wonderful I am, but she's too sensible for that. She's still humming that same song when I return to the kitchen. I'm determined not to be the first to speak. I shall maintain the hurt and pious look on my face, which makes me look a bit like Anthony Andrews.

'I promise I shan't mention it again,' Mum says after a longish silence. 'But I have left you out the *I Love Wholemeal! Diet* on the bed in the spare room. You can do it once you've had Baby.'

My mood remains fairly grim as Mum takes me through the latest goodies she's looked out.

'Ah, now that's the Derekot. It folds away neatly. Terribly useful when you're travelling. They were all the rage in the early sixties. Katie used to sleep in that under the pear tree in summer!'

It looks about as foldable as a Transit van.

'And what about these?' I'm holding up one of a pile of rigid, plasticky shorts.

'Playtex Party Pants. Those were yours, darling, and you looked quite a picture in them! They were from the Tiny Deb range.'

'And did I wear a lot of stuff from the Tiny Deb range, Mum?' I'm squirming now, really praying that I didn't.

'Only for parties and coffee mornings. Oh, I'd forgotten about these!'

As Mum talks excitedly about the Bunnykins tea set, I rummage through a whole stack of old knitting patterns with little darlings modelling the clothes on the front. They simply don't make babies like that these days: over-fed emperors with waxen faces, jam-pot cheeks and flaxen hair, stuffed tightly into woollen suits. They smile and seem to look above the camera, towards the future. Note to self: really must learn to knit. And sew. And crochet. Oh yes, and make lace, embroider, do tapestry and possibly install a loom. Good for making family ponchos.

We set out after lunch to do some errands in town. Mum is insistent on buying me a new maternity outfit. When I confess to her that I have been wearing these dungarees pretty solidly since month four she literally tries to wrestle them off me. A bit of a tussle ensues with me laughing so much I think I'm going to have an accident on the kitchen floor.

As we walk and talk alongside her little shopping basket on wheels, she simply won't be drawn into too much detail about her experience of childbirth. Katie was born at the end of the fifties and I was born in 1968. She tells me that she had my sister in a maternity home and me on the NHS. And that's that.

'But what was it *like*?' I pester. We've just stepped into the butcher's, a high-street abattoir with a ripe smell of blood and large hinds of flesh being hacked up in front of us.

'What a place to discuss childbirth!' she says.

We look at each other and laugh.

'Can't this wait till we get home?'

Once we've got the tea brewing back home it's time to look at our purchases. Mum managed to frog-march me into the Mum's the Word boutique and persuaded me to take a long flowery skirt and large cardigan. I didn't have the heart to protest, she was so delighted with her choices.

'You see, those darts are really cleverly placed. And that elastic at the back will give you room to manoeuvre right up to the birth. And the cardigan's super.'

The cardigan is not super. It has gold blazer-buttons and slightly padded shoulders.

'Shall I take the dungarees off you? I could make them into nice neat rags for Dan.' Mum is the only woman I know to have neat rags. 'I'm sure he'd love them for working on the car.'

'So come on,' I say encouragingly, 'what was the whole giving birth thing like in those days?'

Mum sniffs slightly and stirs her tea. 'It was absolutely fine, dear. Your father dropped me off and I was there with the nurses for ten days or so. Dad was very good about visiting and bought me lots of lovely Yardley things. And there we were! We had a lovely bonny girl to show at the end of it.'

'Come on, it must have been painful?'

'I don't really remember. I was so enraptured with you babies that I really have forgotten about any pain.'

'Mum, don't get all Joan of Arc with me.'

'I really don't see why your generation make such an awful fuss about it. Think of Granny – she gave birth under the kitchen table on a pile of newspaper with doodlebugs whirring overhead. You're so obsessed with your insides, you girls, always talking endlessly about your plumbing and your cupboards.'

'Cupboards? What do you mean?'

'You know, your inside cavities. Your ...' Poor Mum can barely get the words out of her mouth.

'Mum, by "cupboards" do you mean the uterus?'

Mum's face glazes over with concern and she avoids eye contact. 'You see, there you go, talking in that awful way about your monthly activities and tubes.'

'But isn't it better to be honest and upfront about it, rather than cloak it in mumbo-jumbo?'

'The biggest mistake we have made, and there have been many, in the second half of the twentieth century, is talking about everything. In my day we were too busy to talk. We got on with life. Instead of all this mithering.'

There's no stopping her, she's on a roll.

'All you're interested in is yourselves, your generation. You want it all and you want it on a plate. You've had it so easy, you bunch of lily-livers!'

'Mum! I can't believe you're saying this! Kate and I have worked hard, haven't we? You're proud of us, aren't you? For having some sort of career and financial independence?'

She thinks about this. 'Well, I do wish Kate hadn't been arrested quite so many times. Thank God she's through that ridiculous anti-nuclear phase. And as for you, well I do wish you wouldn't drop your aitches when you're on the television, but yes, of course I'm very proud of you.'

She gets up from the table and starts to hum a piece of light opera and prepare supper, her sign that the conversation is well and truly closed.

I can see I'm going to have to work harder if I'm going to get anything other than 'cupboards' out of her. I adore my mum, but I want the truth. I'm going to need some help and the only person I can call on is a certain Señor Domecq. Mum's tipple has always been a nice dry sherry before supper and I conspicuously leave a generous glassful next to the cooker. While she's busy with the meat cleaver, I top up her glass. She starts to hum that little bit louder as we tittle-tattle about local gossip and family.

'Well, I am enjoying myself!' she says, brushing down her apron with the tiniest hint of a slur in her throat.

Glass three is poured while she clatters around in the larder for a bouquet garni. She drops a whole jar of herbs and laughs out loud.

'I shall have to be careful! Too much rummaging in my cupboards could damage my health!'

Bingo. I know I'm on course now.

A couple of glasses of red wine at the dinner table and Mum is well and truly there. Her normally immaculate hair is looking slightly lopsided over one ear, and she has a bright red spot of colour on each cheek.

'I feel very gay I must say! *Prost*!' Another slug of vino goes down the hatch.

'Have some food, Mum.' I'm getting a tad worried now. I've suddenly got an image of her roaring round the streets singing *Iolanthe* and vomiting into a bin.

'Must phone Dad!' she says. 'Must phone him and say *Labas!*' (Lithuanian for 'cheers' and another indelible sign of how far gone she is.)

I attempt to steer her back to the subject of childbirth, before it all gets too messy.

'So, Mum, I was born at lunchtime, wasn't I?'

'Yes. Just had time to put my cigarette out, I seem to remember, before the whole thing kicked off.'

'And what was it like?'

She looks around her, leans in towards me and whispers conspiratorially into my face, 'Ghastly. Utterly ghastly.'

This is all going very well.

'I tell you what, you can get hold of some really super drugs these days. And my advice to you is,' and with this she points a slightly off-beam finger towards me, 'take them all. Whole damn lot of them. All I had was some sickening gas and then it was one long hideous opera of pain.'

On the word opera she rolls her eyes like a diva. She's on fire.

'And what's more, I was so badly depressed after having you that I didn't even want to pick you up. I kept saying, "Take Belinda away from me! Take Belinda away!"'

'Belinda?'

'Yes, I was so brain-buggered I couldn't even remember your name!'

This revelation is a shock.

'But, Mum, you felt better after a bit, didn't you?'

'Oh yes, right as rain. But you listen to me, if you feel strange or low, then you just talk to someone. It can be a dreadfully lonely time just after the birth. And I was lucky. I had two au pair servants to help.'

Two? Full respect. This I never knew.

'And I'll say this,' she shafts an enormous sluice of red wine into her empty glass, 'a lot of child-rearing can be very, very boring. There, I've said it. Bloody boring. Love you two to bits, some marvellous moments. But my God, the coffee mornings!'

She's beginning to enjoy herself.

'Go on,' I beg her.

'Remember Mrs Quail?'

I have a vague memory of being taken to a tweedy suburban lady's house on a few occasions.

'Quail was an absolute pest. Thought she was the first woman to have given birth. Thought she knew the answers to everything: "George is speaking already and he's only eight months." Then: "George's potty training is so advanced blah-di-blah." Urgh! My darling, all we ever heard about was George the Podgy Prodigy. And you know what he's doing now, her beloved George? Works in a petrol station! Ha!'

I feel it's time to manoeuvre Mum upstairs to her bedroom. She carries on as we waddle up the stairs together.

'Quail was a cow! And her petrol station son is a hoyden! I hated those silly coffee mornings. They were simply excuses for the women to bore each other about how marvellous their children were. Never go to a coffee morning.'

'I promise I won't.'

I stretch her out on the bed now and take off her shoes and she offers her final words of the night: 'Quail was a bitch!'

And with that she sparks out. I sleep with the dungarees in my bed. I wouldn't put it past her, even in her advanced state of inebriation, to creep up and have them off me.

105 days to go ...

MUM SEES ME OFF AT Leatherhead station in full tweeds, the county look somewhat marred by the addition of an enormous pair of seventies shades. Her voice is as delicate as a Royal Doulton tea service and I notice that her hands quaver over her ticket at the parking machine. But even in her almightily hung-over state, she's put together a package fit for a boarding-school gel off on a train to Mallory Towers: a ginger cake, homemade mint sauce, four tea towels, a Tupperware box of Bolognese sauce, some carbolic soap for Dan and various cuttings from the garden. She's trussed together the ancient baby equipment with some rope. So much for the Derekot's foldability – it's big enough to sit in and get a tow home. Sitting here in the train I look like a war evacuee. Just throw in a gas mask and I'm ready to go.

Mum slams the train door, which makes her wince and hold her fragile temples. She looks sheepishly through the lowered window.

'Let's not tell Dad about our little snifters last night.'

'Mum, I wouldn't dream of it! Thanks for a lovely time, it's been brilliant.'

I feel sudden tears welling up. This could be the last time I see Mum before the birth. She pokes a finger gently into my chest.

'And I'll make sure that I come up to London and see you at least twice before the birth. I've got lots more things for Baby. There wasn't even room for you to take the mackintosh mattress, for goodness' sake.'

Ah. My tears stop in their ducts. I should have known I wouldn't get away with it that easily.

The whistle blows, the train moves out of the station. There is just enough time for Mum to shout, 'And don't eat mangoes! Baby'll end up as hairy as Helena Bonham Carter!'

98 days to go ...

FOURTEEN SHORT WEEKS TO GO until D-Day, and we still haven't managed to sort out the Pawel issue. Dan did try to tell him while I was at Mum's, but he's been very elusive of late. If you're very lucky you catch the briefest glimpse of him streaking through the front door, a flash of corduroy and carrier-bag bursting with academic papers.

'Look,' I suggest to Dan, 'let's tell him together. It'll be much easier that way. We'll sit him down and just spell it out very simply that he's got to vacate his room by the end of this month at the very, very latest.'

I'm feeling unusually adamant for what has been a very spongy couple of weeks. I've been trying to spend the time 'tidying up before the baby's born'. This involves shifting piles of stuff from one part of the flat to the other, sometimes moving stuff between piles to make them look slightly different, and building up smaller suburbs of mini-piles around them because they look neater that way.

My fingers have now become so sausagey that I had to remove all my rings before the flesh grew up around them, enclosing them for ever. It was all very James Herriot. I soaped up my hands with Fairy Liquid while Dan tugged and grunted till they slipped off. Not only do I have fishmonger's hands, my double-chin is so big my face looks like it's resting on a half-inflated hovercraft – combined with the copious amounts of gas being produced at my rear-end, I could easily provide a daily service to Calais.

This is the week that my sister's kids are coming to stay with us while she and Jake go off for the weekend. They'll be with us for two whole days and a night in between.

I nip down the high street for a special kiddy-based supermarket shop and it suddenly feels like a dry-run for the real thing. Soon it'll be our little one who's demanding cartoon character yoghurts, cheesy dipper things and chicken nuggets. Gone will be the days of one basket between the two of us – it'll be trolleys with those big plastic cars attached to the front of them. We'll finally be able to park in those big Parent and Child spaces that we've looked rather envyingly at all these years.

I am determined to be a serene mother in the supermarket. Not one of those frayed husks slapping the backs of my child's legs. I will not howl abuse at them down the breakfast cereals aisle, and I will really try not to appease their tantrums with goods straight from the shelf. Patience and calm will be my code words. I will glide like a Bloomsbury Lady down the aisles. People will look at me and shake their heads in admiration.

93 days to go ...

IT'S MID-MORNING and the merry beep-beep of my sister's Renault 4 announces that they're here. We haven't seen each other for months and Kate's amazed at how big my bump is.

'Oh my God, look at you!' she keeps saying, feeling its dimensions. My niece and nephew – Tom and Jessica – tumble out of the car, with bed-heads and shy faces.

'Look, sweetheart! What's inside Auntie Mel's tummy?'

Tom thinks about it for a bit. 'Peter Pan.'

'Sorry, he's obsessed.'

Tom lifts up his right arm to reveal a large hook where the hand should be. It's been made out of coat-hanger wire and covered with silver foil.

'Look at my hook,' he says proudly.

'That's great, Tom!' says Dan gamely.

'I'm not Tom,' he retorts sharply. 'I'm Captain Hook.'

'Yes,' explains Kate, 'he won't respond to anything at the moment unless you call him Captain Hook.'

'Right you are, Captain Hook! Ahoy there, me hearties! Arrrrh!' With a swashbuckling manoeuvre, Dan and Tom leap into the flat in search of crocodiles.

Little Jessica is trailing a mangled rag of old blanket behind her and looks ridiculously cute with big marble eyes and bob haircut. She's a very sweet and affectionate two-year-old, and comes forward for a completely unselfconscious hug. It feels great. Her hair smells like hay and her little body clings koala-like to mine.

'Juice? Juice?' she pleads.

'Come on then, let's go inside for a drink, shall we?'

We all sit drinking tea at the kitchen table while Kate and Jake give us a rundown of the final checklist.

'There's loads of stickers, crayons and cut-outs to keep them amused. Tom just loves making art,' Kate says proudly.

Tom and Jessica are like two cubs nestled up on the sofa together watching the *Peter Pan* video. I look at them and beam. The room looks so complete with two children in it. There's a scary quantity of clobber for their one-night stay – it looks enough for a good-sized foreign holiday to me.

Kate and Jake are nearly ready to hit the road.

'Now, are you sure you're going to be OK?'

'Of course!' we protest in unison, and then Dan says, 'Just get totally hooched, enjoy yourselves and forget you ever had kids.'

'This is so kind of you. Now what've we forgotten? Oh yes, we're trying not to give Tom sugary or e-numbery things because he starts bouncing off the walls.'

That's most of my supermarket stuff off the menu then.

'If he needs a snack then I usually just give him a dried apricot. Let him go to bed with the hook on, but take it off once he's asleep because he tends to swipe himself with it in the night. Oh, and he's scared of the hoover.'

'That all sounds fine,' says Dan. 'And what about little Jessica?'

There is a tiny silence as Kate and Jake exchange the briefest of looks. Jake says, 'Well, she's two.'

'Yes?'

'They can be a bit funny at that age.'

I glance over at Jessica who's giggling with delight at Tinkerbell waggling her little fairy bottom.

'She'll be great,' I say. 'Look at her!'

Kate seems a trifle uneasy. 'If she gets moody or shouty, just ignore her. Oh, and always put her down to sleep with Blanky.'

'Blanky?' says Dan blankly.

'You know, her comfort blanket,' I say. 'Like I had my Ubby. Remember Ubby?' I ask Kate.

'Urgh! That disgusting stinky old hanky you used to suck! How could I forget.'

'And what did you have, Dan?' I cajole.

'Come on,' I say.

He coughs. There is a pause.

'I had Ian. Made him out of Meccano. Slept with him till I was twelve.'

It's time for them to go. They avoid big drawn-out goodbyes to the kids, who are too engrossed in Never-Never Land to notice. Dan and I wave Kate and Jake off by the car.

'I forgot to say, Jessica's scared of the bath-plug,' says Jake out of the window.

'Oh, and there's her potty training,' adds Kate. 'She's basically got the hang of it but take extra knickers for her if you go out – just in case. If she needs to do anything she'll say "pot-pot".'

We nod wisely.

'You are total stars. See you tomorrow evening! Any probs, give us a call on the mobile.'

'Uncle Dan and Auntie Mel will have the situation well in hand,' I say, sending them on their way with reassuring levity.

Note to self: must get some dried apricots.

Peter Pan finishes and we've got an hour till lunch. Jessica's first cry of 'pot-pot' has been safely answered with pot and pee meeting in perfect synchronicity in the hall. She trots off to play with her dolly. What a little darling. Tom demands to see the rest of the flat, so I take him upstairs with me while Dan gets their lunch ready.

It's bang on midday when both announce that they're hungry – these kids are like clockwork! Dan's ready with lunch, and then Jessica's ready for her afternoon kip. Bingo! She's out like a light in her travel cot hugging her Blanky. We've put the two of them in our bedroom for the night and the two of us are going to camp down in the living room.

I have the self-satisfied glow of a mother who has done her chores as I descend the stairs to find Dan and Tom deeply ensconced in a conversation about Captain Hook's eating habits. Tom's so questioning of everything, it's wonderful – his little untarnished brain is like a sponge for information and chat.

'I think Captain Hook ate haddock,' Tom announces.

'What about baked beans?' says Dan.

'No. Hook can't eat baked beans cos you need two hands to open a tin and he's only got one hand cos he's Captain Hook.'

I decide to join in from the sofa. 'What if he took off his hook and attached a tin-opener instead?'

Tom ponders this for a second. 'No. He's Captain Hook. Cos actually if he had a tin-opener he'd be Captain Tin-Opener and he's not. He's Captain Hook.'

Dan and I laugh. I feel like we're in an episode of *Little House on the Prairie*. Who needs Playstations and DVDs when you've got autumn sunlight streaming in through the windows and a clever little nephew to make you realise how simple and beautiful life can be?

Kate said that Jessica always sleeps for an hour and a half after lunch, and unbelievably, on the dot of two o'clock, exactly ninety-one minutes after I put her down, we hear her chumbling in her cot upstairs. She's bright-eyed and rosy-cheeked after her kip and once the two of them are watered, we pile Jessica into her buggy and all set off for the park. We're singing a rousing version of 'One Two Three Four Five, Once I Caught A Fish Alive!' as we go down to catch the bus. Other passengers smile fondly at our little family unit, singing its merry way to the park on a sunny London day.

It's three o'clock and we arrive at the park. Dan and I have never actually seen the playground area before. It's been tucked away at the far end of the park all this time and we've never known or cared about its existence. Wow! There's bouncy tarmac flooring to land on and lots of things to clamber up, whizz round and slide down. The sun has gone in, making it a tad chilly, but the kids are scampering around like a pair of hares. A text message comes through from Kate: 'We've arrived. All OK?'

I text her back: 'Wonderful. Beautiful autumn. Heavenly kids.'

I'm finding it hard not to be lyrical.

Dan and I sit on a bench and oversee proceedings like proper, real live parents. The last time I sat on a park bench I smoked fifteen Rothmans and snogged a boy called Jason who carried a flick-knife. I wave at Tom. There he is, swinging his hook around on the roundabout. Jessica's a bit further off digging in the sandpit.

'Isn't this great?' I beam, patting my bump.

Tom bounds up to us. 'Snack, please,' he demands forthrightly.

Of course I forgot to buy any dried apricots.

'Let's wait for snacks, Tom.'

'Captain Hook.'

'Sorry, Captain Hook.'

'I can't. I'm huuuuuuuungry,' he says, stamping his foot like a little bull.

'Come on, Captain, be a good boy,' laughs Dan.

'Not Captain!' Tom says churlishly. 'Captain HOOK!'

Dan rootles around in his pocket and pulls out a dog-eared chocolate bar. Tom's eyes expand to double the size and he starts to jump up and down.

'Yeah, yeah, yeah, yeah! Choccy, yeah, yeah! Choccy, yeah, yeah!'

'Maybe not, Dan. Remember what Kate said?'

'Look, it's not going to do him any real harm. Parents get so worked up about sweets and stuff. Anyway, he'll work all the energy off in the park.'

Which makes total sense to me. Anyway, we're in temporary charge of them, so we have the right to make a few little decisions.

The chocolate has an immediate and startling effect, like somebody doing poppers on the dancefloor of an eighties' nightclub. Tom roars off in the direction of the roundabout. As Dan gets up to patrol him, I notice that Jessica has started to cry in the sandpit.

As I approach I'm greeted with the wailing sound of 'pot-pot'. She must have been calling for it but we were too far away to hear. Not only have we forgotten to bring the potty out with us, there are no spare knickers either. And there was me congratulating myself smugly as I left the house because I brought juice and toys with me.

Poor Jessica. The pee has soaked through her knickers, tights and jeans. The chill in the air has turned into a positively sharp wind, which has started to slice across the park.

I hear a shout from the roundabout where Tom and another little boy are both crying. Dan's talking to the boy's dad – oh dear, there must have been a fracas.

Jessica is a little too heavy for me to pick up at this stage of my pregnancy. The bump has actually started to ache if I lift things. But I have no choice here; Dan's got his hands full over by the roundabout. As I heave her up towards me I feel a sharp pain descend into my nether regions and a tepid dampness spread over my stomach as my niece's wet tights mark her special territory all over my tummy. I'm not quite sure what to do. I can't take all her clothes off; she'll freeze to death. Jessica's starting to cry in earnest, her mouth is now shaped like a letterbox and she's settling in for a good one.

'Ssssshh, my little Jessica! It's OK, Auntie Melly's here.' I try to soothe her. 'Now let's balance you on this litter-bin,' huge wailing now, 'and take your nasty wet knickies off. And trousies. And tighties.'

What the hell's happened to my usage of the English language? Note to self: must never ever say 'tighties' again.

I manage to pin her to the top of the litter-bin and rummage around in my bag at the same time, which involves a sort of principal boy-in-panto lunging manoeuvre. This is going to play havoc with whatever's left of my hamstrings. I have nothing to cover her up with, so I unwrap my rather nice cashmere scarf from around my neck and create a sort of dotee for Jessica, up through the legs to limit any more leakage, and around her waist like a little sarong. I bundle the wet clothes into the bag, dampening my Filofax and lipstick. Jessica does not like her new woollen skirt one little bit and starts to wrench at it.

'No, Jessica. Keep skirty on. Look! Here's dolly! Nice dolly!'

I plonk her into her buggy still wailing, and wheel her over to Dan. I need safety in numbers.

It turns out that, high on chocolate, Tom took a swipe at the little boy on the roundabout and literally gave him a very sharp left hook to the jaw. He has a bright red welt to show for it. The father wears earnest vegetarian shoes and has graphic designer stubble to match.

'Look, that hook could have someone's eye out. I think you should get him to take it off.'

'We're really sorry, aren't we, Tom?'

Tom screams that he's Captain Hook and jumps up and down tearing his duffel coat off.

'Come on, Captain Hook,' I cajole, 'let's take hooky off. It's a bit dangerous. Say sorry to this poor little boy. We can put it back on at home.'

This little speech has a truly terrible effect on Tom. He proceeds to lie on the tarmac and scream. Vegetarian dad backs away, holding his son by the shoulders and shaking his head. He's probably thinking what terrible parents we are to give a dangerous weapon to a hyperactive boy, and to allow our daughter to go semi-naked in freezing weather.

We are the unwelcome additions to a truly crammed bus of shoppers on the way home. Everything's so unwieldy. Between wails, Jessica demands to be carried, so the buggy has to be dismantled for us to get on board. You need some sort of qualification from NASA to work out these buggies. There's a whole sequence of levers to press before you have to lean your whole weight on to the contraption while pressing on a hinge to flatten it and thus render it portable. The bus driver's starting to get really impatient, as poor Dan wrestles with it on the pavement.

'Push the thing on the side!' shouts a passenger trying to be helpful.

People are looking at Jessica's woolly sarong with pity in their eyes, and two teenagers whisper into each other's ears and stare at us. I feel like telling them to eff right off. I am bright red in the face and my hair looks like Ken Dodd's.

'For God's sake, hurry up, Dan. This is really embarrassing!' I shout over Jessica's wails.

Some helpful biddy near the front says, 'She's hungry that one!'

'No, she's not,' I snap back. 'She's fine.'

'Maybe she's cold? Look at her poor little legs, she need some tights on a day like this.'

'They're covered in piss so I took them off, all right?' I'm shouting at her now.

'Piss is a rude word,' says Tom sadly.

'And you be quiet as well, Tom.'

'Captain Hook,' he says defiantly, 'and why hasn't Jessica got any knickers on?'

'Because I forgot them,' I say through clenched teeth.

'Why did you forget them?'

'Because I'm six months pregnant and my brain is like bloody semolina.'

'Bloody's a rude word. It stands for "By the name of our Lady", which is actually even more rude.'

Jessica has gone momentarily quiet, which is a blessed relief, and her face has a faraway, concentrated look to it.

'Why do you always say rude words?' pipes up Tom. I suddenly feel the urge to slap him on the back of the legs. Supermarket Serenity Lady flashes before my eyes. How different she is to this red, growling mess that I have become in the bus. There is a pungent smell emanating from my cashmere scarf, which is still encasing Jessica's bottom. The little tike's crapped into my cashmere!

She takes up the wailing where she left off and Tom comes out with the words we really don't want to hear – 'I want my Mummy.'

Oh no. It's like a magic password unleashing the floodgates. Tom crumples and reddens and Vesuvian tears jet forth. Jessica joins in too. If you half-shut your ears they're like a very cutting-edge modern shouty choir.

'Mamma! Mamma!'

'I want Mummeeeeeeeeeeeeeeee!'

Rows and rows of people are now looking at us as if we're child-abductors.

Where are the parents of these poor little mites? they're thinking. Why has that poor little lad been forced to wear a hook? Look at the mottled cold legs of the little girl! Quick! Call Esther Rantzen!

I don't know how we make it home. The journey feels like it has lasted for a thousand years.

My bump, calves, knees, eyeballs, scalp, brain, fingers and shoulders are really aching now. I'm exhausted and all I want to do is sink into a warm sea-salty bath and take the weight off everywhere. No chance.

'Look, it's not my fault I forgot her knickers. We've both got to take responsibility for things like that.'

'Kate had the knicker discussion with you, Mel. Not with me.'

'Well, what about the chocolate? I told you not to give it to him!'

'He's over it. Come on, he's fine.'

Actually Tom has forgotten about Mummy and has settled down nicely with a piece of toast and Marmite in front of *Peter Pan*.

'Don't make a mess there, Captain Hook!' I say with a rather hysterical laugh. Too late. He drops it Marmite-down onto the rug.

Jessica starts crying again. I go over to offer a cuddle, but nothing seems to soothe her. I take her into the kitchen for a sing-song, but my lusty rendition of 'Lavender's Blue, Dilly Dilly!' falls on unreceptive ears. She doesn't want food, she doesn't want drink, so what the hell does she want, for Pete's sake? Me to dance a naked Lithuanian jig in front of her with celery sticking out of my ears? I'm so distraught I might just do that. Oh please God, all I want to do is put my feet up on my own in a quiet room, listen to some light chill-out music and watch some mindless entertainment on the telly.

Meanwhile, Dan is trying to save the rug from the toast assault. He's a good man. Not a lot of blokes even know where the cleaning equipment is kept, let alone how to use it. But very soon the sound of Tom screaming is drowning out the sound of the … Oh no!

'NOT THE HOOVER!' I yell. 'HE'S SCARED OF THE HOOVER!!'

Tom scarpers into the kitchen ashen-faced and stands screaming by the ironing board. I can see his larynx wobbling. I have truly entered Hades.

Somehow the clock has crept round to five-thirty – I've never known a clock go so unutterably slowly – and it's nearly suppertime. Tom's hoover jitters have been calmed, although he will not under any circumstances go anywhere near the living room now, not even up to the door. Jessica's crying has mutated into a low-level drone, and her jaw has started to judder.

'I don't know what to do,' I wail to Dan. 'I've tried everything. She won't eat or drink or be comforted in any way.'

A pause.

'She wants Blanky,' says Tom.

Now why didn't we think of that? Of course, out of the mouths of babes, oh blessed, wise little Tom!

'Blanky? Blanky?' I say brightly to Jessica. The first smile we've seen all afternoon crosses her face and the relief in the room is palpable.

'Blanky Blanky Blanky!' she says, truly contented.

'I'll get Blanky!' says Dan.

'It should be in the basket underneath the buggy.'

Thank God, my cosy curl-up on the sofa's not looking so distant now. Maybe with a nice little mug of hot chocolate.

Jessica is getting quite insistent and has started a mantra of 'Blanky? Blanky? Blanky?' at quite a loud pitch. No sign of Dan or Blanky. Her mouth is starting to form itself into the letterbox again. Come on, Dan! Hurry up! He sticks his head round the door.

'Blanky? Blanky?' says Jessica.

'Blanky? Blanky?' I say.

'I'm afraid I've drawn a blanky. I mean a blank.'

'What?'

'There's absolutely no sign of bloody Blanky anywhere, I've looked everywhere.'

'It's definitely not in the buggy? Underneath?'

'No.'

'In her bed?'

'No! I tell you I've looked everywhere.'

'She'll have a tantrum without Blanky,' chips in wiseguy Tom.

'Just shut it, Tom!' I snap.

'It's Captain Hook!' he says, mortified, lip trembling.

'No, you're not, you're Tom. Now just put a sock in it, will you?'

I suddenly have an image of myself, sleep-deprived and greying, walloping him in a supermarket. This afternoon's experience has made me realise what an incredibly short journey it must be to get to that stage.

Tom starts to grizzle. Urgent action is needed before Beelzebub and all of his helpers are unleashed into this flat.

'I know! I've got a great idea!'

I waddle upstairs as quickly as I can and fetch an old T-shirt from my wardrobe. It's old and cuddly and hasn't been washed for ages. Perfect.

'Here's lovely Blanky!' I say proudly as I force it into Jessica's flabbergasted face. But the girl isn't fooled for a second. This is a Blanky impostor. She hurls it to the floor, follows it rapidly with her own body, arches her back and screams as loudly as teenagers being shunted round by skinheads on a waltzer. This is a scream to wake the dead. This is a scream to bring our neighbours shuffling round with the police. Dan's face has turned a grey-blue.

'I told you she'd have a tantrum,' says Tom, shaking his head sagely.

Just as Jessica's screaming reaches its top peak, who should walk into the kitchen but Pawel. He seems completely unperturbed, bows slightly at the door, goes to the fridge, gets some ham from one of his waxy packages and a glass of lukewarm tap water, and then slides out of the room again.

'Do you think we left Blanky in the park?' shouts Dan.

'Oh God! Do you think so?' I reply at the top of my voice.

'Must have done. It's nowhere in the flat. You'd better go and have a look for it, Mel.'

'Me? Me!' I shriek. 'I'm six months pregnant, for God's sake. I can't just go into a park at dusk!'

'Well, what would you rather, look round the park or stay here with Hook and the harpy?'

I leave the car beside the park, which is now a cold and desolate place. It's quite a walk through spooky avenues of trees to the playground. Parks are very bleak, I decide. I envisage one of those yellow police boards up on the pavement: 'Heavily pregnant woman last seen in this park searching for Blanky. Found chopped up into small pieces (woman not Blanky). Did you see anything? Phone Crimestoppers.'

I shiver. It's getting very sinister now. The roundabout looks like a hulking beast lurking in the darkness. I hear a loud creak and practically jump out of my skin. The swing has moved for no apparent reason, as if the ghost of a child were on it. I say a Hail Mary under my breath. It's amazing how I can suddenly revert to Catholicism in moments of need.

I look everywhere – sandpit, swings, slide, all the places we went with the buggy. I even venture up and down those morbid darkened paths again. It is nowhere to be found. I sit on the bench that Dan and I had sat on only hours previously, proud as pigeons as we surveyed our domestic scene, and now look at me – a worn-out mess of a wannabe mother and I've only been doing it for seven hours. We have made the biggest mistake of our lives. I want to turn back the clock right now. I don't want to have a baby. It's rubbish having to look after kids – all they do is wee themselves, demand things rudely and then scream for hours on end. I want to be somebody else. I want to be Pen! It's Saturday night – she'll be freshly showered, made-up and dressed in an understated yet groovy way. She'll be with interesting media friends in a Soho watering-hole sipping some newly invented cocktail, before hitting a Notting Hill house-party, full of fizzing wonderful people with lots to say about their fulfilled, drama-packed lives. Compared to old fat-arse here, freezing her lady-nuts off on a park bench looking for a scrap of rag. I phone Dan in floods of tears on my mobile. But it's no good, he can't hear a word I'm saying because of the screaming in the flat.

Right, I need to call on the strength of my Lithuanian forefathers here. I am not going to be defeated by a blanket. It's a simple matter. Blanky is in this bloody park somewhere and I shall find him. (Or is it her?) I am not going back into that hell-hole which is my home before I do.

An hour later and my humour failure has turned to hysteria. I have started talking to myself in that slightly deranged way that whiskery women do in shopping centres.

'Blanky, yes Blanky, he's a naughty sausage, isn't he? Where can he be? Oh dear! What can the matter be! Little Blanky got stuck down the lavatory!' I sing. Then I laugh unhingedly. I have scoured the entire area. Blanky has done a Lord Lucan. We'll have to give Jessica a sedative. Or we'll just have to call Kate and Jake and get them back from Shropshire. That's what we'll do. All pride has gone. I just need to lie down now. It's just as I'm losing all hope, I see a flutter of material underneath the roundabout, as if it has been twisted round and round the damn thing. Closer inspection proves that it is indeed an oilier, slightly more tattered version of Blanky. I carefully untwist Blanky and I lift it high above my head like the FA Cup. I kiss it and sniff it as if it were a family member that had been missing for months. Time to go home.

The park is really dark now, and I have to keep a pretty steady rosary of prayers going as I head towards the gate. Which has been locked. My unwieldy little pregnant legs can in no way attempt to mount it or the fence which runs away on either side. With not one solitary passer-by around to help me, I dial 999 on my mobile. A comforting voice asks me to choose the emergency service I require. I'd quite like all three at this juncture but I plump for the firemen.

'This is terribly embarrassing but I've managed to get locked into a park. I think I need one of those winch things that you use to get cats out of trees. But I'm a lot larger than a cat. I'm six months pregnant, you know.' Of course, just as soon as my call is put through, the heavy rusted gate slides open with unfathomable ease. Not really locked then. I make my unconvincing apologies to the fire service and hurry home with Blanky held tight beneath my arm.

Poor Dan seems to have wizened to the size of Mother Teresa in my absence. Jessica looks like she's been on heroin for all of her two years and Tom just looks very, very depressed. The effect of Blanky on Jessica is incredible though. One sniff of it and she's fast asleep, a little smile curling round her lips. Dan bundles her into her cot straight away. One down, one to go. I might just catch the end of the evening film. Tom pleads and pleads to watch *Peter Pan*. With the afternoon we've all had, dammit I'd give him a collection of Fabergé eggs if that's what he wanted. We all settle down to watch it for the third time of the day.

I receive a text message from my sister: 'Pissed! Brilliant party! All OK with you?'

I switch my mobile off before slumping in front of the scene where Peter Pan fights with his shadow.

92 days to go ...

DAN AND I SLEEP HUGGER-MUGGER on cushions downstairs. After a few hours I shun him in favour of a large pillow stuffed between my legs to combat the calf cramps, which have me up and howling. With that and my now standard three nocturnal loo-trips I am finally beginning to understand what the 'wee hours' actually means.

Peter Pan and Wendy fill my dreams. They are on a roundabout, whizzing round faster and faster. Wendy's wearing my scarf and cackling maniacally. Suddenly it becomes trapped, Isadora Duncan-style, around the spindle of the roundabout. It starts to wind tighter and tighter round her neck so that she's choking, eyes bulging and her face blue. Meanwhile Peter Pan's done a large pee so that there is an enormous wet patch in his green tights. It's starting to spread all the way down his legs. Wendy's not laughing any more but staring at me like a gargoyle with a big black hanging tongue. Peter's pee is forming a lake around his bootees, Wendy's dying, I can't seem to reach the roundabout, I've got the concrete waders on again, I can't reach her, I'm drowning in Pan's pee, oh help me, somebody help me ...

'Can we watch the video of *Peter Pan*, please, Auntie Mel?'

I wake up with a shudder. Two little figures are framed in the doorway. It's still dark outside.

'What time is it?' The crust around my mouth suggests it must be some ungodly hour. Positively satanic – the clock says 5:50 a.m. The kids clamber on to our cushiony mess, happy, sprightly and frisky. How can they be so fickle? What about yesterday? It's as if the traumas never happened. They are ready for the new day, yippee! I, on the other hand, feel like an old pumpkin that has had its insides cored, de-seeded, mashed, pulped and turned into soup. The *Peter Pan* credits are soon rolling again.

I can't believe it's only 7:20 a.m. Time is moving excruciatingly slowly. We've exhausted another screening and the kids are now leaping around in their pyjamas, demanding hide and seek, games and chasing. Dan's digging deep into his resources, making Tom squeal with laughter by turning him upside down, but my humour glands are totally dry. I am seeing through gravelly eyes and want to crawl into a bath with a huge balloon glass of brandy. Kate and Jake aren't due back for another eight hours! Eight hours in Kiddy Time. That's like ten weeks Greenwich Mean Time. How in the name of God are we going to fill them? I know one thing, I'm going to make damn sure that Jessica, pot-pot and Blanky are never far apart.

Somehow time passes. We manage to see the other side of midday using a combination of the *Peter Pan* video (three more viewings), Dan making a den out of the sofa cushions, and me orchestrating a very cunning game of Sleeping Lions where I am the lion and am always asleep – I keep that going for a good hour.

I know what emotion Brian Keenan must have felt as I see Kate and Jake, our very own hostage-release team, roll up in the car outside. Oh happy, happy freedom. I feel a momentary surge of energetic love towards the kids and make a rather lame stab at the hokey-cokey. Kate and Jake look rested and well, like they've been away for a week, and having looked after their children for a night I can understand why.

'How was it, guys?' they ask.

I'm about to respond with a soothing blanket of diplomacy but Tom gets there first.

'Auntie Mel, you see, actually shouted at me in the bus so Jessica was crying and didn't have no clothes on. And then, you see, the hoover was actually very, very scary and Blanky was gone away and Auntie Mel was saying rude words all the time.'

We all laugh merrily at Tom's little speech, I the loudest and rather too hysterically.

Dan and I are lying in silence on our bed after I have tried unsuccessfully to soak my cashmere scarf in detergent. It's with a heavy heart that I admit defeat and bag it up for the rubbish-men. Exhausted, we have lost the power of speech. And there's still all the ruddy tidying up to do. After a weekend with the two terrors our flat looks like a student squat. Cheesy dipper debris is everywhere, the carpets are trashed with trodden-in spittle and biscuits, the windows are smeared with tomato paw prints and, the most perplexing mystery of all, we find Dan's shaving kit covered in flour and neatly packaged in a sock at the bottom of the wardrobe.

There is a lot to take on board. We lie, each engrossed in our own thoughts.

'Let's make the most of the next few months,' I say dourly.

'I now understand why fathers have that glazed, depressed look in supermarkets,' says Dan. 'They are simply trying to block it all out. They just need a space, a little green, breeze-filled space to float in, somewhere above the gunge.'

I nod. 'I now realise why I never see any of my friends who have kids. It's because they are prisoners in a living hell.'

A pause.

'Dan?'

'Yes.'

'Do you think we've made the most monumental mistake of our entire lives? Right now I want to run away to the sun and live childless and free for the rest of my life.'

Dan thinks about this. 'It was bloody funny that you rang nine-nine-nine.'

I laugh. A bit at first, and then I am rattling and shaking with laughter. Dan's caught it too. Hysteria has infected our weakened bodies. I try to stop but once one of us tries to stop the other starts, and we end up in a cycle until I think I'm actually going to vomit. I have to haul myself into the bathroom, but even then we carry on laughing through the walls.

85 days to go ...

THERE SUDDENLY SEEMS LIKE a hell of a lot still to do. No, let me rephrase that. We have done nothing. There is everything to do.

I start with a list of essentials: clothes, nappies, bath, pram, toys. There are more confusing items too. 'Muslin squares!' the sensible lady doctor says in her book, as if she were imparting the long-lost secret of the pyramids. 'You must have them in plentiful supply.'

Then there's the car seat, the bouncers, the bumpers, the knockers, the bottles, the gizmos, the sterilisers and scourers. There's the baby monitor that you rig up so that you can listen to the little one. We'd better get one of those, even if only to monitor what our friends at dinner parties are saying about us behind our backs. Not forgetting the fleeces, blankets, sheets, undersheets, Moses basket and squeaking things. The rain gear, the snow gear and the suncreams. The bath toys! We must have floating things! And what about my bag for the hospital? The midwife said that I'll need pads of all descriptions – everything leaks apparently. And paper knickers! And energy tablets. Six nighties (that's what my mum insisted) and something to make you smell nice. A bowl of pot pourri maybe? And some presents for the midwives. And something to wrap the baby in as soon as it's born. Swaddling stuff? What do you need for swaddling? Something furry? Oh and slippers, I must have slippers and some eye masks. And I need a rocking chair – every new mum must have a rocking chair. And some nice lipstick. There'll be visitors in hospital and I'll need a nice coral colour. And a comb. And plenty of hankies. And did I mention muslin squares? Then we need a jolly frieze in the baby's bedroom. Something farmyardy or circusy. And a nice nightlight and some locks. We must, I repeat must, get locks all over the house: locks for the loo, cupboards and sockets. And a cat-proof net to put over the cot. And what about medicine? Babies are always catching bugs. We must have the necessary pills, potions, gripe-water, thermometers, snot-busters, inhalers, nappy rash cream and probably more pads. WE MUST HAVE PADS!

I think I'm getting stressed again. I lie down with some biscuits in front of an old episode of *Lovejoy* to calm down.

80 days to go ...

WENT SHOPPING YESTERDAY in an attempt to put a serious dent in the To Do baby list. I came home with just two items: a very pretty lamp on a delicate glass base and the entire *Thorn Birds* saga on video.

I started off with good intentions, heading for Babyworld, list in hand. Babyworld is located between Leather Planet and Universe of Sofas, on an industrial estate delicately misted in fumes from a nearby flyover. I'm assured it will be my one-stop shop.

'Hi, welcome to Babyworld, we're here to help!' chirps a young sales assistant, wearing glittery deely-boppers to complement her pastel acrylic uniform. 'Old Macdonald Had a Farm' is playing on the tannoy loop. Babyworld workers smile at regular intervals, their uniforms crackling slightly in the manufactured warmth.

I walk down the Baby Hygiene aisle and become breathless with stress at the amount of nappy choice in front of me. Super-absorbent or midi-flow? Pull-up, foldback or tie-down? His or hers? And a special organic green pack called Back to Nature. I witnessed Jessica's excrement – trust me, there was nothing natural about it. The other aisles offer no simple solutions either. My trolley remains empty for the entire hour that I traipse around this over-lit, air-conditioned nightmare. I am surrounded by other mums-to-be, smiling at each other weakly in sensible, stretchy clothes as the enforced jollity of the tape continues its piercing journey. 'Row, Row, Row Your Boat' has just rowed around for the fifth time.

It's finally too much. I take a seat in the shoe department to gather my thoughts, surrounded by the accepted everyday hysteria of children trying on shoes. There is just far too much ... gubbins, that's the word, in this place. Call me old-fashioned but when I was young I didn't need wind-up underwater musical gizmos, I had a flannel to play with. And my room wasn't a gew-gaw-filled Mecca to Disney and Barbie. I had flowery wallpaper and a poster of the *Blue Peter* gang, thank you very much. My wardrobe wasn't bulging with fake fur coats, angel wings and mini-tiaras. I had one gingham dress and lots of warm, sensible hand-me-downs. We're being duped into spending squillions on tat for our little tyrants. And frankly, my child shall grow up in dungarees, with a flowerbed and some old bowls and spoons to play with.

Another helpful assistant, who must be moonlighting from her local comprehensive, approaches me.

'Have you seen the special offer on the baby-wipes warmer, madam? The wipe reaches baby's bottom electrically pre-warmed.'

Oh God, please get me out of here. I feel the life-force being sucked from me. I leave my trolley where it is and make a break for the exit. I shoot past a revolving Wendy house and cover both my ears to block out 'The Wheels on the Bus Go Round and Round' while simultaneously singing a Clash song as loudly as I can. As I reach the door I'm approached by a happy assistant peddling the Babyworld Clubcard. I collapse into the car, pull the door shut and stare blankly at the dashboard.

75 days to go ...

THE WHOLE ISSUE OF OUR BABY'S inner life has been on my mind for the last few days. That and video four of *Thorn Birds.* I've spilt a lot of daytime tears recently over it. There's something about falling for a priest which I find unbearably moving at the moment.

I've decided that if I am to enrich my baby's inner life then it is time to face up to something, and it is very harsh. I don't know anything about anything. When I was sixteen my brain was in pretty good shape: I won a Balloon Debate and I had poetry published in the school magazine.

I think working in daytime television has rotted my brain, memory and thirst for knowledge. Trivia sticks all right. I know which skin exfoliant J-Lo uses, how Dale Winton managed to lose all that weight, the breed of Lorraine Kelly's dog and what it eats for breakfast. But I know nothing remotely important. I'm haunted by the embarrassment of being grilled by my children.

'Mum, how does a volcano work?'

'Er ... it's a sort of very hot mountain and ... when the mountain gets cross it goes "Whoosh!" and fire comes out.'

'Where does the fire come from?'

'It comes from the centre of the earth which is very hot.'

'Why is it hot?'

'Because ... er ... it's to keep us warm.'

'So why does it get colder in winter? Do volcanoes go to bed?'

'Sorry, dear?'

'Mum, who was Oliver Cromwell?'

'Ask your father.'

* * *

I've decided to expand my knowledge. I'll make a virtue of it and treat it like cramming for an exam. My mission is to revive as much basic, useful, general information as possible, to pre-empt the questions that trouble young minds: Where does electricity come from? Why is sky? What are those doggies doing?

70 days to go ...

THERE'S JUST TOO MUCH to know. Fifteen minutes into the *Pears Encyclopaedia* and I start to panic. Dates of Scottish kings, world populations, land masses, longest rivers, highest mountains, Newton's Laws, the basics of Morse Code, herbs and their uses, the mechanics of the steam engine. Oh, here we go: 'Volcanic activity is caused by the movement of plate tectonics. There are two main types – the andesitic and the basaltic ...' That's the problem with knowledge, much of it's not worth knowing and even if it was it certainly won't all fit in my stewed turnip of a head.

65 days to go ...

I HAVE A NEW PLAN. I'll specialise. Become the sort of mum who knows a hell of a lot, I mean an awful, awful lot, like just about everything there is to know, about one special subject. Before this baby has arrived I shall become an authority in something.

I tell Dan about my scheme. He's in the middle of sanding shelves to go in the baby's non-existent nursery.

'I'm going to become an expert in astronomy.'

I had decided this last night, as I pressed my nose up to the window and watched the first stars start winking in the sky. How infinitesimally small we all are, I thought, how minuscule our baby will be compared to the magical vastness of this great black sky above us. How endless! How universal! And then it hits me. Astronomy!

'Wouldn't it be better to learn Polish? Then you could tell Pawel in his mother tongue to get out of our nursery,' sneers Dan before silently putting his shoulder back to the sanding machine.

Pawel is a meaningless dot against the unending panoply of the skies. Our baby's head is going to be filled with the Big Dipper, the Giant Bear and that Small Saucepan thing. While other children wonder what twinkle twinkle little stars are, you, my little one, will know. The mysteries of the birth of the universe, of life – it all fits. Tomorrow I start my journey to the stars.

64 days to go ...

IN THE BOOKSHOP, I affect a nonchalant, slightly studious air around the astronomy section. I scan the shelf in search of an *Astronomy for Beginners* to get me going, but there doesn't seem to be anything to fit the bill. All the books look rather weighty and dense. None of them has any pictures, just intense little diagrams and hieroglyphic equations.

I approach the owlish adolescent behind the desk with a badge pinned to him telling me his name is Ian.

'Hello, Ian,' I begin with matey confidence, 'I'm looking for an *Astronomy for Beginners* type book.'

Ian, with a distinct lack of mateyness, slides from behind his desk to reveal a body that has no buttocks, and large feet housed in grey slip-on shoes.

'You do mean astronomy and not astrology? It's a common mistake.'

His voice has an irritating, patronising twang and annoys me in the same way that my driving instructor's once did.

'I assure you I know the difference between Patrick Moore and Russell Grant,' I say, trying to retain my zest while simultaneously affecting an aura of knowledge.

'Astronomy's not really a subject for beginners,' Ian continues. He sighs and fingers the books, selecting three or four. 'Do you have a basic grounding in physics?'

'It might have been some time ago, Ian, but I don't mind sharing with you that I was awarded the Marie Curie Prize for Physics when I was at school.'

Ian nods sagely while playing with his bum-fluffed lips.

'Strange that they named your school physics prize after a chemist.'

63 days to go ...

In my embarrassment I'd pretty much taken the books he'd picked without a second glance. They came to £112.50 all in. Astronomical, but it was too shaming to back out.

I sit down today at the kitchen table with the weightiest volume and get stuck in. Good to start with the heavy stuff while the brain's at its freshest.

57 days to go ...

I HAVE CARTED all four astronomy books to the Marie Curie charity shop. I never want to see their turgid little covers or brain-scorchingly dull insides again. They might as well have been in Polish. I couldn't make head nor tail of them. After reading and re-reading the first page of R.N. Barrett's *Laws of Astronomy*, I realised that I hadn't actually absorbed a single sentence. One of the books was full of angles and equations. I feel so stupid. I didn't want maths. I wanted shooting stars and the wonder of the universe. This episode has produced enough humble pie to feed a primary school. I'm so frazzled. It is pointless trying to expand my mind. I'll just concentrate on my talent for expanding my trousers instead. Another ham and cheese toastie, I think.

50 days to go ...

'WHEN DID YOU LAST SEE PAWEL?' I ask Dan this morning.

We rack our brains.

'Do you know what, I don't think I've seen him since the kids were here.'

'But that was weeks ago!'

This is worrying. We decide to investigate. Dan taps on Pawel's door – no reply – and we creep into his room like a pair of naughty kids. Everything seems normal, other than a little bowl of sad, withered fruit on his desk.

'Doesn't look like he's been here for a while,' says Dan, who folds back Pawel's bedclothes and starts sniffing the sheets.

'Dan, that's disgusting!'

'I'd say he hasn't slept in these for a couple of weeks.'

'You don't think he's dead, do you?'

'Let's check the wardrobe,' says Dan, well and truly getting into Columbo mode.

As he gingerly opens the door, I'm fully expecting Pawel's corpse to come thudding out. Thankfully there is nothing, just the usual array of brown and dun clothes. The sleuth in Dan can't resist having a rummage and at the end of the rail, semi-hidden behind some polyester turtlenecks, Dan makes an interesting discovery.

'Ah!'

He holds up several hangers with leather straps and shiny metal rings attached to them.

'What the hell's that?'

Dan grins. 'I think we've just discovered what Pawel likes to wear at the weekend.'

'What do you mean, "wear"?' I ask, getting slightly scared. My

Leatherhead sensibilities have always meant that the penny, particularly the sexual penny, takes rather a long time to drop. 'Oh my God!' I whisper theatrically, eventually. 'He's an S&M freak!'

'Hilarious! There's some lederhosen and a whip back here too.'

'No, Dan! Shut the wardrobe. Shut it. Quick. Let's get out of here.'

I'm going to have to get a priest in to exorcise this room before the baby moves in. This is terrible.

'Do you think we should call the police?' I ask Dan.

'Don't be such a prude, Mel! Loads of people are into this kind of thing. When we next see him we've just got to ask him politely to leave.'

That's it. That's definitely it. Pawel is going, Bavarian leather goods and all.

45 days to go ...

My bump is at the stage now where it's being listened to, sized up and prodded by midwives every two weeks. Today is our first antenatal class at the hospital. The literature tells us the class will cover pretty much everything from waters breaking through to delivery, with a breast-feeding workshop thrown in at the end.

We are a motley selection of eager first-timers. About twenty people in all, mostly in couples, except for a thirty-something lady in a beret who is parked quietly on her own. We sit expectantly, in more ways than one.

One jolly woman with swollen ankles smiles at everyone, while her equally jolly partner holds her hand and grins inanely too. She's in a lavender rugby shirt and he's opted for the lumberjack look. It takes about five minutes for them to chum up with another similarly jolly-looking couple. They're dressed in matching his 'n' hers lemon. The women have started to chat loudly about, guess what?

'So when are you due?'

'Early January. How about you?'

'The same!'

'Oh that's great, we might see each other in the labour ward!'

A suffusion of giggles. Then the Lumberjack husband chips in. 'Well, if you don't see each other in the labour ward you'll certainly hear each other!'

This really tickles the Lemon husband, setting off guffaws of bassline husbandly laughter, while the wives giggle away like sopranos. That's sealed it, they are firm friends now. I can see them on holiday together as a jolly foursome with the babies in lavender and lemon baby-gros. How they'll laugh as they tell their children, 'Yes, we all met in antenatal classes, isn't that hysterical?'

There is something about enforced group activity that immediately puts me on edge. On the one hand the innate show-off in me wants to make gags and get everyone to like me, but there is also a dark side that is balking at all this – why should all of us women get on famously just because we're pregnant? The only thing we have in common is distended tummies with something wriggling around inside them. Nothing more than physical coincidence. It's like asking a whole bunch of asthma sufferers to hit it off, or a group of burns victims to get on like a house on fire. I'm annoyed that those two jolly couples have clubbed together so quickly. They've become the class clique before it's even begun.

Our teacher arrives – a senior midwife called Stella. She smiles perfunctorily and takes up position by the slide projector. She has mountains of handouts to distribute, the mere act of which sets off gales of whispering and giggling among the Jolly couples.

'It's a bit like school, isn't it?' says Lumberjack, looking round to the whole class for approval. His hilarious comment has set the wives off again, giggling like morons.

Dan and I are sitting at the back, trying to play it cool. Stella tells us that the first of our sessions is to be dedicated to What To Do If The Whole Thing Kicks Off At Home.

'So, any ideas? What do we do if the waters break at home?' asks Stella.

'Go down the pub!' is Lumberjack's quip.

I nudge Dan's thigh really hard. To my utmost annoyance most of the class laugh, even old Beret-head, who looks like she hasn't cracked a smile for decades. Even serious senior midwife Stella smiles indulgently at this checked oaf of a man. Damn him! He's fast becoming the class clown, a role that by rights, as the only professional performer in the group, should be mine.

Stella sparks up the slide projector and we are shown a series of couples at home dealing with the onset of pain. A man massages his partner's back, another rubs his partner's thighs supportively. Then there's a third showing a woman wiring herself up to a little box.

'This is a clever little device,' Stella informs us. 'It sends tiny electric impulses into your lower back region and many labouring women find it very effective for pain relief. It's called a Tens machine.'

'Shouldn't that be a Tense machine?' says Lumberjack, laughter already building in his voice. 'That woman in the picture certainly looks a bit tense!'

And bang on cue, as deftly as Bob Monkhouse himself, he reaps another laugh from the audience. Stella actually laughs this time. I turn to Dan and shake my head in disbelief.

The last slide shows a woman in obvious pain, immersed in her bath.

'Water is great for pain,' Stella tells us, 'and you might find it helpful during these first contractions to pour warm water over your tummy too.'

She flashes up another slide, showing caring partner pouring jugs of water over smiling woman's pregnant tummy.

'Hey! Nice jugs!' is the comment from Lumberjack. Surely the scales will fall and the class will now loathe this little man like I do? No, the punters are lapping him up.

'Well, we have a comedian in the class!' says Stella, eyes twinkling merrily. 'What's your name?'

'Steve,' says the idiot, loving the attention.

'And your partner is...?'

'Gaynor,' replies the lumpen lavender lady, delighted to have been singled out.

'Well, everyone, Steve and Gaynor should have a ball during their first stages of labour because you know what? Laughter is actually a great pain reliever!'

The class murmurs their approval. I can't believe I'm hearing this. Laughter? I'm not going to be reaching for my collection of Goodies videos, thank you very much, I'll be sending Dan out for heroin derivatives. I scowl at Steve, who looks as though he's just been given the Nobel Prize for Comedy. His chest is puffed out like a woodcock. Stella continues.

'OK, let's move on. By this time, Baby's head will be engaged and should look like this in the uterus.' She pulls out two props from behind her. One is a baby doll and the other can only be described as an Eastern European tea-cosy. This is to be our very own class uterus, lovingly fashioned by someone very deft at crochet. Stella stuffs the doll's head into the tea-cosy and demonstrates what the engaged head looks like.

Stella clicks the slide machine and a picture of two lesbian partners flashes up. Steve lets out a small wolf-whistle and Gaynor elbows him in the ribs, giggling.

'These two partners have decided it's time to come to hospital,' says Stella. 'Mum is dilated sufficiently for labour proper to commence.'

A voice pipes up within me, I can't stop myself, and I say very loudly, 'How very New Labour!'

There, my first little gag to the class. And I think quite a clever little pun it is too.

Dan squirms, crosses his legs and looks intently at his foot. There is a crushing, resounding silence in the room. No smiles from Stella. She looks positively annoyed at the interruption. I feel the distant Siberian winds of my forefathers blow through the room, a soft funeral hymn played mournfully on a balalaika. A hot beetroot flush rises up from my very heart to the tips of my follicles.

'As I was saying,' says Stella crisply, 'the lady in this slide is now ready for labour, and as long as nobody else has anything else to add,' she throws me a look, 'we'll move on to the next stage of pain management.'

After two hours, the session ends with Stella showing us a 'gas and air' canister. Now this I've heard about. Inhale this combo and it'll give you a nice little high to ease you through your contraction. Stella inserts the mouthpiece and shows us how to inhale deeply on it. The device is then passed around the room with everyone looking politely at it. When it gets to Steve, he rams the mouthpiece into his silly gob and starts rolling his eyes around, shouting, 'Nurse! Nurse!' like some appalling slapstick routine from a 1970s sitcom. The class bursts out laughing. Even Dan can't resist a snigger. How can he be so disloyal?

After the class we pass the two couples exchanging phone numbers in the car park outside. The Lemon-heads drive a neat little estate, and Steve and Gaynor have a rather flash Audi.

'Oh no, look, Dan!' I whisper. 'Look what they've done!'

I am appalled to see that Steve and Gaynor have already attached one of those Baby on Board stickers to their back window. They are just beyond smug.

40 days to go ...

I SIMPLY CANNOT LOCATE my pelvic floor muscles. One of Stella's hand-outs tells us the importance of strengthening this particular muscle-group. When she asked us in class last week who had been doing their exercises, everyone but me put their hands up. Even Steve put his hand up, which got Gaynor in fits yet again.

Dan tells me that they're the muscles you use to stop the flow of pee. Apparently they take a hell of a beating when you're giving birth and it can result in incontinence if you don't strengthen them up properly. Oh great, that'll be mother and baby in nappies then.

Stella took us through the exercises, a clenching and releasing movement, and suggested we practise them while doing something routine like driving or watching TV. I'm practising today as I drive to the hospital for a blood test.

I turn left out of our road, into second gear and *clench*. Down the main road, indicate left and *de-clench*. *Clench* round the roundabout, *de-clench* as I change lanes, left turn through the estate and *clench*. Keep it *clenched* for a few minutes, stop at the pedestrian crossing and *de-clench*. I'm feeling a bit dizzy. And *clench* up again as we head down towards the zebra crossing, stop again and *de-clench*. I'm breathless. I haven't done this much exercise in months. I'm starting to grunt and sweat. And *clench*, let the child clear the crossing and on we go, *clench harder* into the car park, and into the space, slowly, slowly, *de-clench*. I lean my head on the steering-wheel to let the faintness pass. I feel as though I've just run a marathon.

The lady taking my blood is called Elizabeth, and her badge shows a Hungarian-looking surname. She has a kindly wrinkled apple of a face with plaits tied on the top of her head like my Polish grandmother. Immediately I want her to take me into her ample Eastern European bosom and cosset me.

As an ice-breaker, I open up with, 'So you're Hungarian?'

This rings a very positive bell.

'Ah yes! Hungary! And you?' She looks at my name on the notes and her eyes mist nostalgically. 'Lithuanian?'

'Yes. Half!' I reply, all coy pride.

'Ah! Vilnius!' she says as she plunges the needle into my vein. 'Such a city! Such a Baltic jewel!'

My blood starts to creep up the syringe.

'When did you come to England?' I ask her, as she whips off one vial and puts on another.

'Nineteen fifty-seven. Ah, my Budapest! We must always remember.' She looks straight into my eyes. 'And your family?'

'My father came here in nineteen forty-seven.'

'Be proud of Daddy! Be proud!' She's pinching my cheeks, which are probably quite pallid by now, what with all that haemoglobin being sluiced out of them. She's got three full vials and is going for another. I start to feel a bit fuzzy round the edges. This and the pelvic floor exertions are making everything go very dark ... very woozy ...

The next face I see swimming before me, I recognise from somewhere. A teacher from school? Slides?

'Melanie!' she shouts loudly into my face. 'Melanie! Can you hear me? Are you all right? You fainted! Can you hear me?'

It's Stella! Poor Elizabeth stands next to her, a picture of concern, holding a sugary drink to my lips and whispering something soothing in Hungarian.

'I'm fine. Absolutely fine. Just got a bit dizzy.'

Stella checks my blood pressure and lets me rest on a nice comfy hospital bed. She gives me the once-over. Here's my chance finally to get in with her and win one over the ghastly Steve in the process.

'Now are you sure you're all right to drive?' she asks briskly.

'Oh yes, I'll be fine.' I lean towards Stella confidentially. 'What is it with the Hungarians and blood, eh? She's the Bela Lugosi of the hospital, isn't she?' I do a little impression of a blood-sucking vampire.

Stella looks at me with a stony contempt. 'Elizabeth has been with us for many years and is one of our most experienced blood workers,' and with that she turns on her heel. Oh please God, somebody make me unconscious again.

38 days to go ...

OUR ANTENATAL SESSION TODAY is no laughing matter and Steve is actually quiet, which is a blessed relief. A man from the council takes the first half of it, and shows the class a gruesome video of car crashes, with tiny baby dummies flying into the windscreen. He's come to show us the importance of strapping your baby properly into car seats, and the whole class is pretty thoughtful and subdued after his departure.

For the second part of the session we're getting physical, as Stella gets the entire class down on the floor and shows us some positions for labour. Our partners have to learn how to help by propping up their pregnant partners, which involves a lot of lumbering, huffing and puffing in poor Dan's case. I feel a pang of sorrow as I clock that Beret-lady has nobody to prop her up. Stella has to play the role of her partner and it makes me brim a bit. Sorrow is subsumed, however, by the humiliation of performing some of these labouring positions. There's one where we're on all fours, like a herd of old mares, and good old Steve soon pipes up with, 'This is what got Gaynor up the stick in the first place!' A big laugh. That's right, we all need a bit of rallying from the class's very own Tommy Trinder. Through Gaynor's legs, I shoot Steve a look of pure venom.

Dan whispers, 'Look at you! It's the Bloke-With-One-Syllable-Name Syndrome again! Remember Jim?'

I don't care what it is, I'd like to get Steve on all fours and grind his gurning face into the ground. As we're leaving the class, Steve sidles up to me.

'Didn't you used to do that thing on the box?'

Good. He's realised that he's in the presence of a professional.

'Yes, Steve, that was me, I'm afraid!' I say modestly. Maybe he's not so bad after all.

'Well, looks like you could do with a hand pepping up your routine,' he says. 'If ever you need someone, I'm your man!'

31 days to go ...

THERE'S ONLY ONE THING FOR IT. Steve and his comedy act must be sabotaged. Every time he opens his mouth now, I cough long and loud to try to block out his stupid jokes. Either that or I greet his every comment with a sigh, a yawn, or a light groan.

The sessions have almost finished, and today it's time for the Big One. Stella is going to show us a video of an actual, real birth.

It all starts off pretty much as you'd expect. Labouring lady starts groaning and is given gas and air.

'Forget her!' says Steve in a reprise of his now classic 'Nurse, Nurse!' routine. 'It's going to be me needing that stuff!' Supportive titters from the men in the group. I yawn ostentatiously.

The poor woman unknowingly evacuates her bowels.

'Yeah, and I'm going to be crapping myself too!' is Steve's hilarious response.

Big laugh, even from Stella.

The labour progresses and the action in the video gets low-down and heavy as the camera pans downwards to the coal-face. As the baby's head starts to appear and the woman's pain worsens with full bellowing soundtrack to accompany it, a truly marvellous thing occurs. In the row of seats in front of me, Steve slumps forwards and clutches his mouth. Vomit is visible from between the cracks of his fingers as he tries in vain to cup it. He runs shakily for the door, moaning. Gaynor goes after him supportively, while the class looks on, concerned. Stella puts the video on hold. There is a subdued silence in the room except for one corner of it. Dan and I are spluttering with barely contained giggles. There must be a God somewhere.

30 days to go ...

'How about Maud?' I suggest.

'Over my dead body. It sounds like morgue.'

We're getting stuck into *1001 Baby Names and their Meanings.*

'But I love it. It says Maud was the wife of William the Conqueror.'

'I don't care if she was the wife of Jimmy Greaves. I'm not having a daughter called Maud.'

'What about Martina?'

'As in Navratilova? You cannot be serious?'

'I am serious.'

'And what if we have a son?'

'Then we could shorten it to Martin.'

'Definitely not Martin. There was a Martin Chapman at my primary school who always smelt of cat food.'

'How about Malvina? It's Argentine for "Falkland Island". That's a bit of a statement, isn't it?'

'The only statement it's making is "My parents are twats". Anyway, why do all of your suggestions begin with M?'

'I'm at the "M" section of the book.'

'Yes, but why? You're just looking for something that goes with Mel, aren't you?'

Dan's got a point. I feel slightly ashamed of myself. I really must try to be a little less self-centred.

'So have you thought of any names?'

'Well, as a matter of fact, I have.'

Dan reaches over to pick up a little notepad on his bedside table.

'Right. For a girl I've got Claudia and for a boy I've thought Galen.'

Silence.

'And?'

'That's it.'

'Those are the only two you've come up with?'

'The baby only needs one name, Mel.'

'Galen was in *Planet of the Apes.*'

'I know.'

'And Claudia Knight bullied me really badly in the Brownies. She pushed me off the toadstool.'

'I know, but I like the name.'

'Then that's really mean of you,' I say, turning over impetuously to my side of the bed. If you can call a slow, heaving roll with two pillows stuffed between one's legs impetuous. 'You're not taking this seriously, Dan. The naming of our child is really important. It's for life, not just for Christmas.'

'Don't joke. This baby could arrive on Christmas Day, possibly during the Queen's Speech.' Dan chuckles. 'How about Santa if it's a girl and Noel if it's a boy?'

29 days to go ...

JUST OVER FOUR WEEKS TO GO and still no sign of Pawel and still no nursery. To add to our load I am staring at a brown patch on the kitchen ceiling that appeared a few days ago. It's damp and today it has started to drip. I've positioned a cereal bowl on the floor to catch the plops of water but the drips seem to be picking up pace.

Mum used to read me the story of Chicken Licken when I was a kid, and I used to find it pretty scary. Chicken Licken thinks the sky's falling on his head every time an acorn hits him, and I have to admit that the kitchen leak is giving me real Licken vibes.

Dan's working in Germany for a couple of days and I decide to take an executive decision. I look up 'Roof' in the Yellow Pages, find the most honest-looking roofer-type person, and get on the phone immediately. (To find an honest-looking firm, select those that have a crest or emblem within their advert. You can't go wrong with a good crest.) Within five minutes I have secured a roofer. He'll be round to give us a quote tomorrow. He's called Bob.

28 days to go ...

Bob the builder arrives bright and early. I resist the temptation of singing the obvious theme tune, but can't refrain from enquiring if Scoop and Dizzy are coming later. Bob ignores this and sets his own agenda.

'What's Brazil's biggest export?'

'I don't know, Bob. Coffee?'

'Thanks very much, love! Milk and two sugars!'

I hope I'm not going to get into One-Syllable-Man trouble with Bob. Must keep my cool. I manage to hum merrily while I make the coffee and he inspects the leak.

'I want a new roof, Bob,' I say decisively.

'Well,' he says, sucking on his teeth the way that all builders do, 'don't think you'll need it. I reckon if we just repair the flashing and patch it up it'll be good as new.'

I have a sudden vision of Chicken Licken, wings flapping desperately as he tries to escape Armageddon.

'I don't want a patch-up job. I need a new roof over this kitchen.'

'When's the Big Day?' Bob says, motioning to my bump rather casually.

'You've got three weeks, Bob.'

Bob sucks his teeth again. 'It's going to be messy and noisy.'

'I don't care, Bob. Just do it.'

'Well, you're the boss.'

I think of Dan and what his reaction is going to be. I might be eight months pregnant, but I must be executive. This is not just a roof, this is going to shelter our newborn from acorns.

'Can you start tomorrow?'

27 days to go ...

EVERYTHING IN THE KITCHEN IS covered with old sheets and Bob plus two Ukrainians are banging away with gusto. They have Heart 106.2 turned up loudly and Bob's doing his best to sing along to 'I Lost My Heart to a Starship Trooper'.

The phone rings. I can just about make out Dan's voice over the banging.

'What's that banging?'

'I've got someone in to sort out the leak.'

'Really? Who?'

'A bloke called Bob I found in the Yellow Pages. When are you coming home?'

Dan is unnaturally silent – I can tell he's worried and suspicious.

'Look, I've got to rush,' he says eventually. 'I'll be back tomorrow about eleven. Don't let him do anything too major.'

By lunchtime they're going great guns in the kitchen. The rotten roof is off and the spaces of sky in between struts of wood are covered with plastic sheeting. It has started to rain a bit, which makes a comforting plopping sound on the plastic sheeting. The Ukrainians look up at the weather and share a private joke in their mother tongue.

It's proving harder to cook than I anticipated with both the fridge and hob surrounded by debris, and all the work surfaces lightly covered with dust. I have lunch in the greasy spoon round the corner and ponder whether my decision-making hasn't been a little too executive.

26 days to go ...

DAN ISN'T VERY HAPPY.

'Couldn't this have waited till I got home?' he says, trying to keep his temper.

'Just what do you think I am? Some brainless, doughy-headed, child-carrying goat? Don't you trust me? Am I no longer Mel? Is that it? Am I just "Mother" now? Have I lost my identity? Have I lost my me-ness? Am I simply a vessel—'

'What are you going on about? Just calm down and tell me how much this is going to cost!'

A silence. My voice is quiet and my bottom lip has started to tremble.

'I don't know.'

'What do you mean?'

'We never got round to discussing it when Bob came to give the quote.'

Dan says nothing, but leaves the house in the direction of the greasy spoon. 'Dan!'

The phone rings. It's Mum. Just hearing her voice at the end of the line makes me dissolve into tears.

'Don't worry, darling! Dad and I will be over tomorrow!'

25 days to go ...

Bob arrives on his own today. It seems the Ukrainians never showed up for their lift this morning.

Shortly after lunch, courtesy of the caff, a shrill voice singing 'Yoo-hoo!' through the letterbox announces the arrival of Mum and Dad. Bob's radio blares loudly, so we didn't hear the bell. Dad settles himself down in the living room with Dan to talk rugby, while Mum heads straight through to the building site to inspect Bob.

'I'm Melanie's mother.' She sounds like the Queen. 'How's it all coming along?'

'We're getting there. What's the main export of India?'

'India?' says Mum. 'I suppose it must be tea?'

'I don't mind if I do. Milk and four sugars, please, love!'

We're soon settled down and enjoying the strains of Bob howling along to 'Lady in Red'.

'So it seems that everything is quite ship-shape,' says my dad, tucking in to one of Mum's enormous flapjacks. He's brilliant to have around at moments like this.

The doorbell goes. It's Mick the plumber. Apparently he's going to re-route some pipes.

'We'll have to turn off the mains, I'm afraid!' shouts Bob through the door. 'Anyone need the khazi better go now!'

Mum opens more packages which she's brought us from home – some Dundee cake, a Tupperware box full of lasagne and six nighties for me, which are all large enough for a group of Boy Scouts to camp in. Mum is offering round the cake when the doorbell goes. Hopefully it's the Ukrainians.

I go into the hall to open the front door and am greeted by three very un-Ukrainian-looking women in sunglasses, one of whom is holding a very large baby.

'Amanda,' I say, rather too curtly to be polite. 'What a surprise.'

'I was in the area, babe! I've started a new yoga class quite near here. This is Anna, my yoga teacher.'

I shake Anna's bony hand.

'And this is Lyn, my fabby nanny.'

I shake Lyn's fabby hand.

'And darling, here he is!'

Lyn holds out Amanda's progeny. I know that all babies are lovely to their parents, and that is the wonder of Mother Nature, but let's face it, there are some real shockers in the pack. Though I'd said he was beautiful in the emotional cauldron of the delivery room, I now have to reappraise. This child has not merely been touched with the Ugly Stick, he has been right royally beaten round the chops with it. He is pushed into my arms and all I can muster is, 'Aaaaaaah! There we are!'

'Say hello to Balthazar,' says Amanda. 'He's *very* advanced.'

With that she swishes into the living room to dispense air kisses. My mum has always been ambivalent towards Amanda, but Dad thinks she's a hoot. He makes her take a seat next to him and sets about entertaining her and her ladies-in-waiting.

Balthazar is about four months old and is so advanced that he can actually look at you with pure boredom in his eyes.

'He's very big, Amanda,' says my mum. 'What are you feeding him?'

'I don't know. What are we feeding him at the moment?' Amanda asks Lyn.

'He's on a high-protein formula.'

'You haven't got him on the Atkins already, Amanda?' I say.

'Oh dear. He'll be obese before he's three,' warns Mum.

Time for more drinks I think.

I head out to the caff for take-out and dream idly of being left alone with *Thorn Birds.* I briefly catch sight of myself and my bump in a shop window and barely recognise what I see. How one stops oneself from toppling over is a mystery.

The party is in full swing when I return. Bob and Mick are on another tea-break and are joining in. Amanda is telling Dad about her planned trip to Phuket. Anna seems to be showing my mum some yoga technique and Dan is valiantly trying to make Balthazar laugh, but is getting no reaction whatsoever. He's probably too advanced for Dan's jokes.

Amanda has very sweetly brought two large carrier bags bursting with Balthazar's hand-me-downs. It's gruesome stuff. Particular horrors are a Bavarian-style skiing jumper with feathers on the shoulders, some jodhpurs and a sailor's outfit made from pure silk. It looks like the wardrobe of an Austrian mayor. I kiss Amanda politely and throw Dan a look.

The doorbell goes again. I feel like we've entered a Brian Rix farce or even *This Is Your Life*. Dan answers it and ushers Jools and little Doric into the living room. It's very sweet really. This bizarrely unconnected set of people has descended on our little flat, sensing that the Big Delivery is imminent, popping in with gifts, good lucks and final nuggets of advice.

Introductions are made. Jools asks for a glass of water, which sadly we can't provide.

'Be back on tomorrow!' says Bob jovially. 'In the meantime you'll have to slash in the garden!'

Bob and Mick show no signs of getting back to work. Mick's chatting up Lyn with risqué tales of his adventures in the plumbing world: '... So I had me face up to the waste pipe, didn't I? Next thing I know my whole head's covered in shit!' He's certainly got a way with the ladies.

Jools opens up a rucksack and hands me a sheaf of papers. 'I thought you might find these useful – some birthing mantras and some beautiful pain poetry too. Henry read them to me all throughout the labour and I found it so wonderful and soothing. My favourite is the piece written by a mountaineer. It's so powerful. It describes each contraction as a mountain that you have to climb.'

Dan and I avoid all eye contact.

'And I thought you might like to borrow this.' She hands me a length of rough material. 'It's a traditional African hessian truss. The women of the Congo wear them during late pregnancy.'

Dan leaves the room suddenly.

'Wow, that's really kind of you, Jools. What exactly do you do with it?' I am faintly dreading her response.

'Well, I couldn't help noticing at Doric's naming ceremony that your belly was quite swollen. If you're expecting a big baby, then this can be tied underneath the bump to help take the strain. It's amazing what you can do with it on. I helped build a local dam.'

A full-throttle scream from Balthazar prevents any further truss-chat for the time being. He starts to whimper.

'I think he might have done biggies,' says Mum.

'No, I don't think so,' says Jools, suddenly leaping forward, kneeling before Balthazar and shutting her eyes. She starts to make a low humming noise and flutter her hands around him. 'With this cry I'm hearing Balthazar tell me that he's feeling confused.'

'I'm sure he's got a poo in there,' says Mum again.

Jools smiles indulgently. 'I've been attending some crying sessions with Doric. It's been very bonding for us. If the baby cries like this,' and Jools throws her head back and does a high-pitched moan, interspersed with short breathless gasps, 'that signifies jealousy.'

The group are frozen, mesmerised by her performance. My dad's got a piece of flapjack up to his open mouth.

Jools continues. 'But if Baby is crying more like this,' and a low gurgle emanates from the deep recesses of her throat, 'then he or she is telling us that he has forgiven us. It's the sound of forgiveness. Whereas this cry,' Jools mewls long and pitifully like a cat, 'means he's probably just resentful.'

There is the unmistakable odour of faeces in the room. Even Jools must be smelling it. Lyn lifts the bellowing Balthazar out of the room to change his nappy.

A rather red-faced Jools says, 'Well, it's probably a mixture of forgiveness, confusion, and *also* poo.'

Mum looks rather smug. 'You're another one with a whopper baby, Jools! What are you girls giving them these days?'

Jools flinches. 'My breast milk's very rich because our goat's on a pulse-based diet. Oh, I almost forgot!' She reaches into her rucksack and brings out a covered bowl. 'I made this for you, it's highly nutritious and great for softening the walls of the uterus.'

Dad's starting to look a bit peaky and has put down his flapjack. Mum is speechless and Dan, who has now returned, looks positively scared, memories of Jools's placenta canapés haunting him. What on earth could this red, jelly-like substance actually be? Jools's own uterus lining? Something that came out of the goat?

'It's jam!' Jools explains. 'Made with quinces from our birthing tree.'

Balthazar has rejoined the group with new nappy. Jools has unleashed one of her enormous mammaries to feed Doric, giving Dad the cue to hare out of the room with the excuse that he needs the loo.

'No water I'm afraid!' says Mick the plumber, who seems to care not a jot about the waterless house, but is helping himself to a large piece of Dundee cake instead.

'I'll use the garden!' shouts Dad on his way out of the door.

And then the doorbell rings again. What is wrong with it?

'I'll get it!' says Dan, leaving us ladies to chat and Bob and Mick to ogle Jools's gigantic breasts. She's started to hum to Doric as she feeds him. I can't put my finger on the tune but it's definitely Lindisfarne's back catalogue.

'How long do you plan to … do that for?' enquires Amanda, looking aghast at Jools's knockers.

'I'll see how he gets on. Obviously it'll get difficult when he starts going to school.'

'But he'll be four, won't he?'

I have a terrible image of poor Doric in a little blazer and shorts suckling on his mother's pendulous baps through a hole in the school fence.

And then Dan enters the room with Pawel. Throughout his entire time as our tenant, I have never been so pleased to see Pawel enter our flat. He's brandishing an enormous bottle of Zubrowka vodka and looks positively healthy.

'Pawel's been in Poland all this time!' announces Dan.

'Please,' says Pawel bowing, 'where is Father?' He and my dad have always got on well.

'He's out in the garden trying to avoid Jools's breasts, which I must say is quite a feat.'

'Mum!' I hiss.

'I go to give him this,' says Pawel, lifting the vodka like a trophy, and exiting.

'I really must get going,' says Amanda. 'The night nanny takes over at six and I've got an aerobics class to go to.'

Amanda slips her Burberry handbag over her shoulder while Lyn is left to bundle Balthazar, expensive large-wheeled buggy and assorted clobber into the silver Jeep parked outside. Amanda kisses me absent-mindedly and wishes me luck with the birth.

'Have lots of lovely drugs and champagne, babe, and I'll come and visit you. Actually, it's Christmas week, isn't it? I'm going to be in Barbados. Shame! Still, I'll send flowers.'

I can't help laughing.

And with that, she is gone.

Jools has undocked herself from her son and is putting him back into his papoose. She gives me an enormous hug.

'Now, are you sure you don't need me to be there with you at the birth? I found it so reassuring to have a circle of women around my birthing pool chanting hymns to Gaia. It's so important to have proper goddess time. We all do it for each other. We can do it for you.'

Dan's eyes are as large as saucers.

'That's lovely of you, Jools. We'll have a think about it and let you know.'

'Be strong and use the pain as a good release, yeah?'

I'm worried she's about to go into her repertoire of birthing screams, and Mum's rolling her eyes, so I hug Jools hurriedly and take her and Doric to the front door. She places her hand on my forehead and shuts her eyes for a moment.

'Gaia smiles on you, Mel.'

Just Mick and Bob to deal with now.

'So, Bob and Mick! The kitchen's ready for you!'

Bob sucks his teeth, looks at his watch, and looks at Mick. 'We'd better get down the DIY shop before it closes. Got a bit of wadding to get.'

'Now where's your father and that scrofulous Pole?' asks Mum, when they've gone. 'He needs to be told that it's time for him to pack his bags and vacate my grandchild's nursery.'

'Er … Mum. Do you think that's really a good—'

But she's already marched out of the back door.

We find Dad and Pawel sitting on a wheelbarrow having a lively discussion in Polish. The vodka level's gone down by a couple of inches, and both are drinking it out of mugs. Dad's chuckling and both of them look very misty-eyed.

'Pawel was just telling me a very funny story about his uncle in Lvov.'

'Never trust the wool of the priest!' says Pawel emphatically, to explain the anecdote, and this sets the pair of them off laughing.

'Now, Pawel,' says my mum, sounding like a primary school headmistress. She's also speaking at twice her normal volume, something which she always does when translating her views to foreigners. 'As you know my DAUGHTER IS PREGNANT! She will SOON HAVE HER BABY!'

'*Sto lat*!' says Pawel, lifting his mug in a toast.

'It is VERY IMPORTANT THAT you listen to me, Pawel.'

I can feel my bowels starting to contort with shame. Dan is looking intensely at the bird feeder on the garden table.

'YOU MUST LEAVE THIS PLACE. IT IS NOT YOUR HOME NOW. DO YOU UNDERSTAND?'

Pawel is smiling blissfully and nodding.

'My dear,' Dad says quietly, 'I've already explained to Pawel, very clearly, that Dan and Mel are sad but that he should vacate his room as soon as possible, ideally tomorrow, so that they can prepare a room for the baby.'

I want to hug him long and hard.

'Oh. Well. That's very good then. JUST AS LONG AS YOU KNOW, PAWEL—'

'It's all right, Mum,' I say gently. 'Come on, let's all go and sit down and have a drink inside.'

We slump in the living room. Dan puts on a little gentle music. Finally I can put my feet up. What a hectic afternoon. Dan fetches three more cups and Pawel makes a toast.

'My preferred English family! And long life to baby!'

'And to your NEW HOME, Pawel!' says my mother tartly. 'Wherever it may be!'

He smiles enigmatically.

Dad says, 'I've said that Pawel can come and live with us ... just until he finds his feet.'

20 days to go ...

'There are some lovely Arabic names. How about Muhammad?'

'I don't think we can lay claim to any Islamic heritage coming from Leatherhead and Huntingdon as we do. You've become very grandiose since you've been pregnant,' says Dan, tweaking my nose rather patronisingly.

'Well, at least *one* of us cares that our baby gets the right name.'

I turn to read my book. There is a pause.

'How about Jordan?' says Dan.

15 days to go ...

BOB'S DOWNSTAIRS, putting the roof felting in place. The kitchen still looks like one of those awful war-torn houses. The job's been delayed with all the rain and now it's a sprint finish between him and the baby. I'm upstairs getting dressed.

I'm now so large that even putting on a pair of knickers takes time, forethought and effort. I've developed a clever routine. First I sit on the side of the bed and throw the knickers down on the floor at my feet, hoping that'll they'll land with the two leg holes relatively open. If they land in a closed position I have to start again with a new pair, which means there's usually a large pile by the bed. Dan hates this and refers to it as the Tracey Emin effect.

I'm on form this morning. The knickers land perfectly so that I can place my right foot in the appropriate hole. Part two of the operation is to jiggle my right leg up with knicker safely hooked above my calf, allowing me to reach them with my hands. Then comes the technical bit. The left foot must be dropped into the remaining leg-hole. If done too sharply or too swiftly, cramp can set in, tears ensue and the knickers are dropped. Then it's like snakes and ladders: back to square one. A softly-softly approach is best at this stage, and I find a bit of light grunting helps enormously.

Once both legs have securely met both holes, then a roll backwards on to the bed with legs hunched up completes phase three. Then a roll to the left to hoik them up over the left hip, followed by a hoik to the right to secure the other side, and the whole operation is completed. I'm pretty efficient now. Like Roger Bannister I've got the whole thing down to under four minutes.

Dan's been beavering away on Pawel's room this past week, and an aroma of fresh paint has replaced the rather musty bachelor smell. We've opted for a custard yellow on the walls, it's supposed to be a good sleep-inducer for Baby.

'How about giving me a hand painting the skirting boards?' says Dan, as I moon uselessly around the baby's room.

'I wish I could, but I have to be really careful of the fumes. Especially gloss paint. I think I'll go back to sewing my muslin squares.'

I say 'go back to' – I haven't actually started them yet. I saunter downstairs, there's a *Juliet Bravo* day on UK Gold – I might just catch a couple of episodes before I settle down to some sewing.

Mum phones halfway through my sixth *Bravo*. Apparently Pawel's taken over my old room. I hope he's not sleeping under my Holly Hobby duvet.

'He's a very nice boy,' Mum tells me. 'Awfully good at chopping logs.'

'That's great, Mum.'

'And I see from all his leather tack that he's a keen horseman. Well, at least he'll have more opportunity for riding here than he would have done in London. How wonderful to have an equestrian in the house!' Mum is delighted.

10 days to go ...

BOB DISAPPEARED yesterday afternoon, saying something about going to St Albans for a special bonding product. It appears that Bob's bonding product must have been very strong indeed, because he only made it back from St Albans this morning. He looks exhausted, red-eyed and there's more than a backsplash of booze on him.

Dan is at the end of his tether.

Luckily I can escape from the house. I've got a midwife's appointment. I'm not saying I'm a coward – I just can't bear any nastiness or confrontation. I blame it on the pregnancy.

5 days to go ...

THE MIDWIFE TELLS ME THAT the baby's head is down and nearly 'engaged'. Which means it could come at any time now. If the baby's more than fourteen days late, a common occurrence with first pregnancies, then I'm told it will have to be induced. I'm given a 'How to Get Labour Going' handout and sent on my way.

As I'm leaving the maternity unit, I hear a familiar jovial laugh bouncing off the walls. It chills me to the core. As I walk down the corridor my worst fears are confirmed. There they are, waiting for their appointment, as merry as two gnomes – Steve and Gaynor. They're in matching velour tracksuits, clasping hands, and Steve is holding court.

'Apparently they put you in stirrups – they'll be using a whip as well: oo-er!'

Gaynor nudges him in the ribs and giggles uncontrollably.

Now surely this cross-section of the great British public will look deep into their psyche and make the decision not to laugh at Steve? Surely they have some taste?

The whole corridor rips up with laughter.

I keep my head bowed down and head for the car park.

Dan's on his own in the kitchen when I return home. He's looking up at the roof thoughtfully, chewing on the end of a pencil.

'Hi!' he says lightly.

'Hi, darling,' I say, taking off my coat. 'Where's Bob? Gone for another long lunch?'

'No.'

'Where is he?'

'He's gone.' Dan turns to me. 'I've sacked him.'

'*What*?! But we've got no kitchen roof and the baby's due in five days!'

'I'm in charge now. It's up to me to put a roof over our heads.' God, I love it when he talks macho.

'It just needs finishing off. Nothing I can't manage. It's going to be fine. Don't worry.'

I can't say I'm convinced, but we now have to pull together.

'Oh, and what's the main export of St Albans?'

'Special bonding product?' I suggest.

'Cheers, love. Milk and fifteen sugars!'

4 days to go ...

DAN WAS UP AT FIVE THIS MORNING and by five-thirty was already up on the roof. It is stair-rodding down with rain, and, as I watch him through the bedroom window, he cuts a pathetic figure in drenched cagoule and plastic trousers. He has propped up the roofing book he found at the library under some clingfilm, and is teaching himself how to put the slates on as he goes along.

The baby's room is pretty much finished now, and the '*layette*', as the baby's stuff is rather unpleasantly termed, is in place. I therefore have plenty of time to peruse the induction handout with a cuppa. The first suggestion makes me splutter out a mouthful of tea. This is the first time I've been ordered to have sex by a quasi-governmental leaflet.

Sex, a warm bath, curry and reflexology are the leaflet's suggestions, in no particular order – a great night in for me and Dan under normal circumstances. But now. Oh dear no, not sex! Are they sure about that. In my current state, what they're suggesting could actually contravene the laws of nature and physics. I try to recall exactly how you go about that. I seem to remember it involves a bit of dinner, wine, and smooching to Lionel Richie. No. That was someone from a past life, a time when I could lift my legs up higher than two inches.

I lay subtle hints to Dan throughout the day, just as fast as he's laying rain-soaked slate roof tiles in his spectacularly unsexy yellow cagoule. By 9 p.m., I'm lightly oiled up and in bed, waiting for him. I've brushed my teeth and puffed up my hair a bit. At the last minute I put on some old fancy dress tiger ears for that sex kitten look. The lighting is atmospherically low so that all you can make out in the room is the vague outline of duvet over my bump, giving the impression that there is a large beer-bellied bloke in the bed. Dan is still tapping away on the slates with the aid of a small torch. I hear him swear occasionally. By 9.05 p.m. I have sparked out. Sex is definitely off the menu tonight.

3 days to go ...

I'M WOKEN IN AN EMPTY BED still wearing my tiger ears to the sound of slate-tapping and it's only 7 a.m. Dan is getting obsessed with the roof. He's started to stroke it lovingly and refers to it as 'she'. He also refuses to come down for lunch, so I have to winch him up a few sandwiches in a little basket.

After lunch I leave him hammering and muttering, and head out for my reflexology appointment. The reflexologist is a very gentle, fragrant man called Theo who sets to work on my feet like a baker making a cottage loaf. I feel sorry for the guy, and not a little ashamed for myself, because I haven't been able to get near my feet for the last five months and I'm sure that the nails have started to curl up like a pair of Aladdin's slippers. He repeatedly massages the pressure point on the foot which represents the uterus.

When I get home I barely make it to the loo before a vicious onslaught of the trots ensues. Seems like Theo marginally misjudged that pressure point, but has done wonders loosening up my alimentary canal. Perhaps this is a sign though. I check my bag and go to bed certain that something's going to happen tonight.

It does. Dan wakes me up around midnight to tell me excitedly that 'the rubberised bitumen's working a treat. It goes on so smoothly it's incredible.'

2 days to go ...

TODAY I TAKE THE SPICE ROAD. I kick off with a chicken madras for lunch, and brave a vegetable phall for supper. It has absolutely zero effect, other than making my other option, sex, utterly out of the question.

1 day to go ...

MUM RINGS THIS MORNING to see how things are going. She says she always did some vigorous gardening to get things moving.

'And darling!' she adds. 'Just one more little thing. Don't paint the nursery yellow whatever you do. Mrs Turton's youngest slept in a yellow room and became a cocaine addict.'

I take up her gardening tip and try to jog and weed at the same time for about four minutes, before collapsing in front of the telly for the rest of the day.

Anyway, there's nothing to worry about. I am never late for anything, never have been, and neither has Dan. In fact, we're the sort of people who arrive at an event half an hour early and sit in the car till it's arrival time on the dot. Our baby is genetically predisposed to do likewise. I can feel it in my waters.

THE BIG DAY

'WHY DON'T YOU BLAST IT OUT with some really, really loud Led Zeppelin?' It's been a while since I've heard Pen's voice – that familiar hung-over croak.

'That's actually not a bad idea, Pen.'

'Try "A Whole Lotta Love" and do a bit of air guitar as well.'

I get the Zep on the turntable and turn it right up.

By evening, esteemed midwives Robert Plant and Jimmy Page have had no discernible effect. Nor have U2 or Wham! Dan makes me a rather weak gin and tonic and I settle into a bath, which is marginally hotter than normal. I feel a bit like a Victorian prostitute using this old gin and hot bath routine.

We take to our bed early and ponder what is potentially our last night of baby-free existence. Life is about to change for ever and there's no going back. I've never experienced anything like this. I thought that leaving home for college was going to be the big life-changer but it was essentially the same, only with more cider. Then I assumed that starting work would be the big one, but I just wore a skirt more often. Meeting Dan was a life-changer, of course, but I've still got my Whimsy collection and he still listens to Fairport Convention so it can't have changed us that much. No, this is the Big One. We are ushering in the next generation. We are moving out of the way and letting him or her take centre-stage. We are taking responsibility for another life. We have created that new life, and with all this comes the overriding whiff of our own mortality.

I sigh deeply. 'Wow.'

'Yeah, wow,' agrees Dan.

'How do you feel?' I ask him.

'Kind of OK,' he says.

'Worried?'

'Sort of.'

'Hmmm. Me too,' I admit. 'It's the Big One, isn't it?'

'I guess so,' he says.

We share the warm, contemplative silence, happily resigned to our fate. Dan turns and looks lovingly, confidentially, into my eyes. 'I'm happy enough with the plastic guttering, but part of me thinks I should have been bolder and gone for metal.'

1 day overdue ...

I'VE BEEN DREAMING OF my mother a lot recently, and last night was no exception. In this particular dream she is on horseback, dressed in leather and carrying a large crop. Every time she whips the horse it lets out a loud whinny. It must be painful. In fact, so painful that it wakes me up. And there it still is, an undeniable nagging pain across my stomach like I've never felt before. I poke Dan.

'Dan! It's coming! I felt it! The baby's coming! Quick, get the bag! It's coming!'

'Let me get the light on. Are you OK?'

'I felt it. A big pain across my stomach. A contraction!'

'Any sign of the waters breaking?'

'Don't think so.'

'OK, let's just calm down and lie here and see what happens. The next one might not be for an hour or more. Want a cup of tea?'

'Yes, please.'

Dan goes to get the tea and I lie, waiting for the next contraction to come. I knew my baby'd be punctual. It's a good sign. Hopefully it'll be polite too and write its thank you letters. Dan brings up our Scrabble set with the tea.

But nothing more happens, other than Dan beating me soundly at Scrabble – he had the audacity to use 'Fallopian' on a double word score. He wouldn't allow me 'Vorderman' even though I'm in labour.

Or am I? Dan read in the sensible TV lady doctor's book this morning that you can get these kind of false contractions called Braxton Hicks.

Pamela Braxton Hicks could be one of mum's old coffee-morning adversaries. And at the moment they're just about as welcome. Can we please get on with this?

2 days overdue ...

RIGHT. I'm going to get executive with this child. I'm its mother and should start to show some authority. I grasp the rubber shower attachment from the taps, put the shower-head firmly on to the bump and begin speaking into the other end.

'Now listen here. This is your mother speaking. We'd quite like you to come out now. Have you got that? The exit is clearly marked and you should make your way there as soon as possible. Please take off all stilettos and use the chute provided. Thank you for your attention.'

3 days overdue ...

'LOOK. THE TINY BABY JESUS managed to do it in time for Christmas, and he only had a stable waiting for Him. We've prepared you a nice room with toys and heating and everything.'

4 days overdue ...

'LOOK, we're not cross. We're just disappointed.'

5 days overdue …

'THIS IS GETTING RIDICULOUS. If you don't come out of there right now your father is going to be very, very angry with you.'

6 days overdue …

'WE'VE GOT SOME PRESENTS FOR YOU! They're all wrapped up round the tree!'

7 days overdue …

'RIGHT, THAT'S IT. No presents. If you don't come out this minute we're taking them all to Barnardo's.'

8 days overdue ...

(SOUND OF LIGHT WHIMPERING.) 'Pleeeeeeeeeeeeease come out!'

9 days overdue ...

'OK. YOUR FATHER AND I are going now, aren't we, Dan? Bye! When you come out there won't be anybody here and you'll be all alone! Bye then! (Sound of door slamming.) You see? We've gone. Nobody's interested in you.'

10 days overdue ...

CHRISTMAS DAY. Dan and I sing in light harmony down the shower attachment: 'Away in a manger, no crib for a bed, the little Lord Jesus lay down His sweet head'.

Then I shout: 'That song is about the BIRTH of Jesus. RING ANY BELLS?'

We've been so absorbed in waiting for the baby that Christmas Day has totally passed us by. We had the traditional Christmas dinner of macaroni cheese, pork pies, toast and chocolate ice cream.

11 days overdue ...

It's Boxing Day and I've given up on the shower attachment. There was a light smattering of snow last night and London looks very restful and white. But I'm thoroughly blue. No position is comfortable any more. Sitting hurts the bump, standing hurts my knees, lying hurts my lungs, crouching hurts my labia. The only relatively comfortable position is on all fours. Humiliating but true.

I feel enormous – having recently switched to a diet of Cointreau-filled, chocolate-covered brazil nuts. I feel useless – Dan's *still* tinkering around on the roof. But most of all I feel bored, bored, bored.

The telly is just rubbish. I scan the paper to see what films are on today. I don't believe it – *Peter Pan*. I'm just settling into it and am tragically joining in with all the dialogue, when there is a crash from the garden. I crawl across the living-room floor and see a figure in fluorescent yellow writhing on the ground.

I bang on the doors and Dan points to his ankle.

'I fell off the bloody roof! Call an ambulance!'

I don't believe this. If there's going to be any ambulance drama round here I'm going to be at the centre of it, thank you very much. I am positively terse with the emergency services.

'Yup, fallen off a roof. Says he's done his ankle in. He thinks it's serious but you know what men are like. Thank you very much.'

Dan drags himself across the garden on all fours, shouting in agony. 'Have you called an ambulance?'

'Yes. What on earth were you doing up there when it's so icy anyway?'

'In case you hadn't noticed, you selfish cow, I've been trying to get the bloody roof done so that our baby is secure and warm. We'd never have got into this mess if you hadn't got that pointless builder in!'

'Oh, it's all my fault all of a sudden? I didn't hear any complaints at the time. But no, let's just blame the poor pregnant lady who can't get up out of a chair without rupturing her spine! I've had nine months of this, nine months of CARRYING YOUR CHILD and I'm bloody sick to the death of it!'

'Oh, it's MY CHILD now, is it? That's right, when something doesn't suit our little princess, she just washes her prissy porcelain hands and walks away from it.'

To an outsider we must look like a pair of Rottweilers, barking and spitting viciously at each other on all fours.

The doorbell goes, and I greet the kindly ambulance men before returning to all fours.

'OK, love. How advanced is your labour?'

'No. Not me. Not the vastly overdue pregnant lady. No no no no no. Of course not, it's my husband. He's through there with a hurt ankle.'

They get Dan onto a stretcher and into the waiting ambulance outside. They very sweetly put me into a wheelchair – which is nice of them.

Dan and I bicker for the whole journey and the poor ambulance man can't even manage to take down our particulars before we arrive at the doors of A&E. Plenty of time once we're there though.

The skeleton Christmas staff try to jolly up their monumentally long shifts by wearing either paper hats or flashing reindeer antlers. The usual array of seasonal injuries awaits them: drunks, festive domestics, a couple of Christmas lights electrocutions, and some unfortunate who seems to have got stuck on a brandy bottle.

We have a five-hour wait in front of us and I intend to ignore Dan studiously. I've had enough. We sit in total silence, looking in different directions.

Suddenly Stella, the midwife, appears out of nowhere, rushing through the A&E door.

'There you are,' she says, starting to wheel me away. 'Can you take any jewellery off before we get you into theatre?'

'Er … I think you've got the wrong person actually. We're in with a grazed ankle this evening.'

'Well, where's my emergency Caesar lady then?' she says and stops wheeling me rather abruptly, leaving me marooned down a corridor.

The lady in question has just arrived by ambulance and Stella rushes off to tend to her. The idea of a Caesarian seems suddenly rather appealing.

Dan is finally seen by the doctor at three in the morning, by which time I am hallucinating with tiredness and Dan's foot has swollen up to the size of a small pumpkin. X-rays show that there is no break, but a severe sprain. The doctor orders him to rest it for as long as possible and discharges him with a pair of NHS standard issue crutches as a memento of his visit.

'Great,' I say grimly. 'Look at us. It's like Ironside and Bob Cratchett.'

They can't stretch to an ambulance home, so we call a minicab.

12 days overdue ...

I'M STILL FURIOUS WITH DAN, who has gathered up almost all the pillows on our bed to rest his ankle on. Every time he moves, his face creases in pain like an injured Italian footballer. One of his eyes has exploded into a swollen purplish colour too.

'Must have caught it on the guttering as I came down,' he says in a self-pitying heroic kind of way.

'Do you want something to eat?' I bark, grudgingly resigned to the ludicrous fact that I am now the most able-bodied of the two of us.

'Anything,' Dan says weakly, like he's been living in a Dickensian poor-house all his life.

I'm muttering to myself around the kitchen like a demented lady-tramp when the doorbell goes.

Bedecked in spanking new sets of Christmas hats, scarves and gloves are Mum, Dad, my sister Kate and brother-in-law Jake, with Tom and Jessica who are reassuringly calmer than last time I saw them. I fall into Mum's arms. She's piled high with Tupperware boxes, tins, cardboard boxes and even a few winter cuttings from her garden.

'We've only come for a bit!' she announces. 'We thought you two might need a bit of looking after.'

13 days overdue ...

NEITHER DAN NOR I have left our bed in the last twenty-four hours. We have been fed, entertained and generally spoiled rotten by my family. Thanks to rest, sustenance and the healing properties of time, we have now even warmed to the funny side of the whole incident.

'I will never forget you, hunched in the garden in that fluorescent yellow cagoule.'

'And I will never forget your humour failure in the hospital by the drinks machine.'

'I love you.'

'I love you too.'

And we switch out the lights. Come what may, I'll be going into hospital to have my baby tomorrow.

14 days overdue ...

WE LOOK LIKE A RIGHT PAIR OF TINKERS, what with Dan's black eye and crutches, and my enormous bulge. We tell the duty midwife at the desk that I've come to have my baby induced, and are logged into the system.

Home, until the baby arrives, is to be the Edith Jones ward. It's a four-person room and each bed can be cordoned off with curtains. We're not quite sure what the Curtain Policy is. If you shut all the curtains then you look unfriendly, a bit off-hand. But if we leave them all open then we feel exposed and won't be able to snoop on anybody, which I am, of course, dying to do. We compromise and keep the side ones closed but the front one open so that the goings-on in the ward are there for us to enjoy.

Dan and I start to whisper to each other. We do it in Bed and Breakfasts when there's only one other couple in the breakfast room, or in very quiet gift shops.

'Did you bring the Scotch eggs?'

'They're in the zipper compartment.'

'What about my refreshing facial spray?'

'It's with the paper knickers.'

'Look, let's stop whispering, shall we?'

'OK. You go first!'

'No you!'

Our banter is interrupted by a midwife who has come to look at my notes and tell us what to expect.

'You'll be given a sweep today and a gel tomorrow morning.'

'I didn't know the hospital had a hair salon!' I say in an ill-judged attempt to entertain, but the midwife crashes on, having seen and heard it all before.

'The sweep is an internal examination and the gel, made from hormones, is placed directly on the cervix, to get the contractions started. If neither works, then we'll break the waters and put you on a hormonal drip the day after tomorrow. Any questions?'

'Is the sweep actually done with a brush?' I ask nervously.

'No.' She smiles. 'Just a hand in a glove.'

'Like Sooty and Sweep,' I say gamely.

'Not a furry glove. It's latex.' And with that she's off.

'Bring on the sweep then!' I say with the bravado of a lacrosse captain.

The word 'sweep' suggests something rather autumnal and ethereal: a serving-girl clad in calico gently brushing the leaves out of a pantry as the fading embers of late summer sunshine reach inside. When referred to gynaecologically, however, the word 'gouge' or 'rummage' would be far more appropriate. When the midwife has 'swept' me, my cervix feels like it's had a platoon of stormtroopers marching all over it. As I'm settling into bed, with my kit all round me, a fresh-faced junior doctor peeks his head jauntily round the curtain.

'Ms Gee-Droyce?' he says, casually mauling my name. 'And how are we?' He flicks through my notes.

'I take it you've been made aware of all the procedures which may take place over the next couple of days?' he asks politely.

'Yes. Thank you.'

He takes my pulse himself. I attempt silence-filling small talk.

'How long have you got to go?'

'A good few years, I hope!' he laughs. 'I'm pretty healthy.'

'No, I mean, before you qualify?'

There's a pause.

'I have qualified.' There is an edge to his voice.

'I see,' I say, 'but I'll be meeting with a consultant at some point, I suppose?'

'I am your consultant.'

He looks like a boy in a doctor's dressing-up kit. I laugh nervously and a little too long for comfort.

'So, if there's nothing you need to ask me,' he says brusquely, 'I shall come and see you tomorrow.' He smiles briefly and leaves.

Dan comes back from the drinks machine. It's eight o'clock and time for him to go.

'Give me a call if anything happens,' he says. 'Are you OK?'

'I'm fine. Or I would be if you could stay here tonight. Can't you break the other ankle?'

He kisses me tenderly on the lips and hobbles off down the corridor.

It's hard to sleep in hospital. The temperature is whacked up to old people's home levels and, never having been to boarding school, I'm not used to the sounds of other women blowing their noses and coughing through the night.

There's a very sassy woman called Alisha in the bed next to mine and I can hear her through the curtain, never off her mobile phone despite hospital restrictions on them. I heave myself over to face the wall and try to get to sleep.

15 days overdue ...

WELL, IT CAN SAFELY BE SAID that the sweep was 100 per cent ineffective. Not even a murmur of a contraction has occurred in the night, so bring on today's dish of the day – a light gel served with a consommé of hormones.

I pull back all of my curtains briskly. I'm in a sociable mood, and even take my breakfast tray to the communal table, hoping that the other ladies in the ward will follow my lead.

'Morning!' I say brightly to an unfeasibly tiny lady with big glasses and a bump which is twice her size. 'Hospital food, eh? It's not exactly Raymond Blanc, is it?'

'She don't speak English, she's from that Albania,' Alisha tells me as she plonks her tray down beside me. She sniffs the milk and wrinkles her nose. 'And this is well off.'

'Do you know what you're having?' I ask Alisha politely.

'A bloody nightmare is what I'm having,' she says, arms folded.

'Oh dear, I'm sorry to hear it.'

'This is my fourth baby in this place. And I can tell you, they don't know what they're doing, yeah.'

'But it's got a great reputation – it's a teaching hospital.'

'Well, they should teach them midwives some manners. They are rude, man. Rude. Look what they serve us!' She points to the cornflakes, yoghurt and apple on her tray. 'It's muck! I wouldn't feed that to my dog.'

It looks OK to me.

'And them beds we have to sleep in? I didn't sleep a wink, man, not a wink. They should change them. And sheets? It's disgusting! No duvets? I'm going to complain. I want my money back, man.'

'It's free.'

'I don't care if it's free. I still want my value for money...'

I leave Alisha complaining to the mute Albanian. I go into my little cubicle and firmly shut all of the curtains.

Dan's arrived and it's gel time. Hopefully this is it now. I look at the clock – 11 a.m. I reckon we should be a three-person family by the time the *EastEnders* theme music starts.

Alisha's on the phone again. 'This ward is disgusting. Full of asylum seekers. And this older woman. She's a snob. "It's a teaching hospital," she says this morning ...'

The gel is put into place and Dan and I decide to take a stroll in the grounds of the hospital – if I hear another word from Alisha I will be forced to suffocate her with her pillow. She'd probably complain to her last breath about that too: 'You suffocating me with this pillow? It's not even feathers. It's rubber. I'm allergic to rubber. It's disgusting.'

There's a real bite in the air today, and a group of crows caw ominously over the prison's exercise yard next door. We tramp around its perimeter slowly, like a couple of old-timers. I'm actually more mobile than Dan at the moment.

Half a mile from the hospital is an athletics track and we decide to head in that direction. We're nearly there when I start to feel a definite twinge. It's like a really really strong period pain. Halle-ruddy-lujah, the gel seems to be doing its job. What I'm feeling is pain relief – actual relief to feel some pain.

'Dan, it's coming, I think!'

'Great.'

'Oooooooow.'

I try to remember the breathing techniques that Stella taught us in the antenatal sessions, but realise pretty quickly that the only thing I absorbed in those classes was a growing bitterness towards Steve and his burgeoning comedy career.

Whenever a woman gives birth in a film, they always do those little tiny gaspy breaths. Vanessa Redgrave did it admirably when she played Wagner's wife opposite Richard Burton. Oh spirit of Vanessa! Be with me now! I attempt a few little gasps, but it makes me feel dizzy. The pain subsides and we make our way over to the track.

Through the railings we watch as a lone athlete hares round the track, breath coming out of him in big clouds of fog. We watch him go round and round for ages, until suddenly I feel another contraction, slightly more intense this time. What was it Jools said? Imagine the pain as a mountain that you're climbing. I concentrate and try to visualise. All that comes to mind is when Mum and Dad took us to the Lake District when I was a kid, and forced us to climb Helvellyn. After a pathetically brief attempt – we whined that it was too hard – Kate and I were left at the teashop at the very bottom.

As we head back to the hospital, finally in labour, Dan holds my hand supportively, but when I start to squeeze it, he howls with pain because of his crutch blisters. What a pair we are.

It's 6 p.m. and after what seems like a lifetime of contractions later, the midwife comes to inspect my progress.

'Can you see the head yet?' I ask her anxiously.

She laughs. 'You're a long way from that, my dear.'

And a latex glove later: 'No, I'm afraid there's nothing happening. No dilation. The cervix hasn't moved at all. I'm going to give you a painkiller and a sleeping tablet and we'll break the waters tomorrow morning at ten.' She smiles with matter-of-fact sympathy and leaves us.

I feel absolutely crushed. Nothing happening? That's impossible, surely. I've been contracting all day!

'Maybe the baby just hates me,' I say, crestfallen. 'Most kids wait till they're fifteen to hate their parents, maybe ours has just cottoned on very early.'

'Oh darling,' says Dan, looking at me through his one good eye, 'don't worry. At least my blisters are feeling better, eh? You can give my hands a good squeeze tomorrow!'

I have never felt so lonely as I watch Dan's stooping figure limp away down the hospital corridor. The painkiller's kicking in, thank goodness, but sadly nothing can block out the pain of listening to Alisha's griping down the phone.

'I tell you what, I'm going to lodge a formal complaint. I was left waiting in my bed for fifteen minutes before anyone saw me today.

Fifteen minutes! Then the midwife tells me to have a bath and gives me a towel that is not even conditioned. It is like sandpaper on my skin. I'm telling you. This is worse than prison in here!'

I shed a few silent tears into my pillow. I have never missed Dan so much in all my life.

We're all woken in the middle of the night by a new arrival on the ward. One of the beds has been empty these last couple of days, and the new resident is already in full labour by the sounds of it. I creep up to my curtain so that I can get a really good look. She's blonde and petite and accompanied by a very solicitous husband, who's probably a solicitor, in cords and brogues. They look posh. Her midwife is with her and is being very encouraging.

'That's great, Tabitha. You're doing really, really well.'

Tabitha moans and whoops in reply.

I can hear Alisha tutting and sucking her teeth behind the curtain already.

'Mmmmmmmmmmmmm, yeees,' moans Tabitha, louder this time.

I shut the curtain and get back into bed. And so it continues. Surely she's not going to go on and on like this? The sound effects are worse than our halls of residence at college. Tabitha doesn't sound like she's in labour, she sounds like she's in the throes of passion, and what a girly swot she is to boot.

'Well done, Tabitha, you're doing brilliantly, brilliantly. You're nearly fully dilated!' coos her midwife.

'MMMMmmmmmmm! Oh God yes!' says Tabitha in a high-pitched squeak, like Kim Basinger in *9½ Weeks*. I hate Tabitha like I have never hated anyone before. She is a perfect prissy little prig and I hate her and her flexible cervix.

Half an hour later and she's still doing the porny soundtrack. Right, that's it. We've been in this ward two days longer than that upstart, and some of us desperately need our sleep.

With the curtains shut I say in a loud voice, very reminiscent of my mother, 'Look I know you're in labour, but would you mind keeping the noise down?'

16 days overdue ...

TABITHA HAD A PERFECT LITTLE BABY at one in the morning. She did it so well that she's been allowed to go home already. The baby's called Jacob and is the perfect weight. I hope Jacob becomes a crack addict and steals from his mother to pay for it.

Alisha barely acknowledges me at breakfast and we sit there in a fug of bad humour.

'I'm not eating this shit no more.' Alisha pushes her cornflakes away and gets into bed.

I lie on mine and wait for Dan to come. Thankfully he's here by eight-thirty – opening time. His eye's gone from purple to yellow. On seeing my downcast face, he says, 'I've brought you some more Scotch eggs!'

Not even that can cheer me up.

'I want to go home. I'm rubbish at this. I don't think the baby wants to come out anyway and it's probably right. I'll be a rubbish mum, I haven't even sewn up those muslin squares ...'

And with that I dissolve into sobs.

'Shhhh,' says Dan, trying to hug me with his one crutchless arm, 'everything's going to be fine. We're going to have the baby today! Think of that! And there have been loads of messages at home for you. And, and,' Dan struggles for good news, 'the roof's holding up really well under these adverse weather conditions.'

I can't help laughing. Dan's eyes are shining with pride.

'She's looking great, and the slates look fabulous with a bit of snow on them!'

'I'm glad about that.'

'Come on, dry your eyes, let's have a game of Scrabble.'

* * *

I somehow imagined that the process of having one's waters broken would be extremely high-tech. I thought there'd maybe be an electronic device or a clever pill.

No.

Valerie the midwife takes a white plastic crochet hook from its packet, approaches the coal-face, inserts it uncompromisingly and pierces away at those ballooning waters.

'Geronimo!' I say rather lamely and high-pitched, as the crochet hook hits home. Dan looks on proudly. His face is rather too close to mine. I hope he doesn't intend to keep it there for the whole of today.

'OK, darling,' says Valerie kindly, 'we're going to take you up to the delivery suite and a doctor'll see you shortly.'

The lift stops on the third floor and a woman is wheeled in on a bed. She looks very pale and on the point of being sick. The doors are about to close when her bloke jumps in. It's Steve. He's holding one of those disposable cameras, like he's on a stag weekend with the lads. He flashes away at his poor wife.

'Say cheese, love!'

He then puts his face close up to hers and sticks up his thumb as he snaps another shot of the two of them together. Please God, don't let the lift break down. We arrive at the fifth floor and Gaynor is wheeled off with her baboon of a husband lolloping behind.

So here we are in this important room which is to be the backdrop for our momentous occasion. But there's nothing memorable about it at all. It's plain and surgical with several monitors and drips, and thankfully a small telly.

Valerie's rigged me up to a monitor and the baby's heartbeat is swish-swishing away.

A young girl with a ponytail bounds in. I expect her to take our orders for teas and coffees, but it turns out she's the doctor. She jabs around to try and get a decent vein in my arm, and then inserts a tap which looks like a bar optic.

'My blood group is Rhesus Vermouth!' I say to the fourteen-year-old medic. She laughs as you'd laugh at one of your grandmother's quips – politely and pityingly.

'All done. They'll start you on the syntocinon drip very soon. If you're going to have the epidural, a lot of women have it at this stage because the contractions come very strong and fast. Good luck!'

'And good luck with your GCSEs!' I can't help saying.

She looks puzzled and makes a hasty retreat.

'How's the pain?' Dan asks, and then winks at me. Something rather odd has happened to Dan during the last half-hour. He has started to wink at me. I think it's the nerves getting to him. It's a sort of cheesy wink that a kids' TV presenter might do at the end of a show when he says goodbye. I look at Dan suspiciously.

'Are you all right, Dan?' I ask.

'Yeah, fine,' he says, and winks at me again.

'I think I'll wait a bit before deciding about an epidural.'

I'm of sturdy Lithuanian stock and I have always reckoned on my pain threshold being pretty high. My fellow Liths would surely have given birth in windswept fields during a brief lull in their potato harvesting. Hand the little one over to grandma, then straight back to the potato digging.

Valerie comes in with plastic bags of fluid and attaches them to the drip. This is weird. I've had nine months to ponder all this and I still have no real idea what I'm about to let myself in for. I just hope it's quick, whatever it is.

She hooks the bags up, takes my blood pressure and then attaches me to another monitor which measures the contractions. There's no escape now. This is what it's all been leading to. The tiny Cheddar-fuelled bug that started off so small is now here, visible, large and waiting to make its entrance. I have chosen my 'Women are Angry' T-shirt to give birth in, and am wearing a rather jaunty bandanna, which will double as a head-tie when my hair gets really sweaty. I watch the liquid from the drip plip, plip, plop into my arm.

Dan switches the telly on for me, and the only channel with half-decent reception is Channel 5. There's a very slushy film with some poor woman being cheated on who keeps wobbling her highly glossed lips.

All quiet on the contraction monitor so far, the little needle just glides lazily across the roll of paper. Then as the lady in the film confronts her lover with the immortal line, 'I had you in the boardroom and the bedroom!' I feel something ominous in my abdomen. It's a pain, yes, but not the sort of pain I've ever experienced. It's not a stabbing pain. It's not a throbbing pain. It's not a burning pain or a bruising pain. This is pure liquid pain which oozes right into your marrow. It comes in ever-increasing waves, and Dan's face is in mine within a nanosecond of its first unbearable ascent. His breath smells of prawn sandwich.

'Give me some space,' I snap at him. Dan answers me with a wink.

Before I know it there's another one of the buggers, which sets the needle off across the monitor like a spider on tequila.

'Do you want a bit of gas and air?' says Dan.

'Yes, pass the mouthpiece.'

Dan proffers the mouthpiece up to my lips but it knocks against my front teeth.

'No! To the left!' I bark.

The needle is now settling into a routine.

'Oh my God, look at that!' I shout as it rides upwards, as if it's about to skittle right off the paper.

'That's nothing,' says Valerie with quiet, disturbing knowledge. 'You'd better just settle in for the ride, darling.'

I don't like the sound of this ride at all. In fact, I want to get off. I'm suddenly reminded of Mum and Dad taking us to Chessington Zoo. I was fearless then – never used to think twice about getting on board that ropey old Alfredo's Big Dipper, which used to shake its rickety way up, up, up so high that you could see Tolworth. That ride had probably never had a safety check in its life. I now feel like I'm back there, perched at the apex of Alfredo's first descent. This is not a good ride to be on, it is potentially lethal and I don't want to be ejected from my seat and spewed out somewhere over the A3.

A few minutes later Dan rouses me from my momentary painless bliss. 'I have to go and renew the parking ticket. It might take me some time.' He looks anxious. 'I had to park quite far away. Will you be all right?' Then Dan's vile prawn mouth is shunted on to mine. He winks and leaves. I can feel another contraction building.

'Go!' is all I can bark, before succumbing to the marrow-twisting pain again.

'Breathe,' says Valerie helpfully, checking the monitor.

I try a bit of Vanessa Redgrave again, but it's totally useless. I want to rip the monitor and drip off, but I can't. I need to walk around and get on all fours or something.

The needle settles down and the pain subsides, allowing me to enjoy Gloria Hunniford's *Open House*, which I've never seen before. Good old Glo. She's looking radiant in camel: 'And today my guest is a close friend. Ladies and gentlemen, put your hands together for Sir Cliff Richard.' Cliff's wearing his trademark blouson leather jacket and waistcoat. His lips can barely contain his teeth as he jokingly tells Gloria about his latest album. Will she join him in a song? They glide over to the singing area, revealing Cliff's moulded showbusiness trousers, patent brogues and Gloria's palazzo pants. They start to croon together. As the song progresses, so does the needle on the monitor. They hit the chorus and the needle peaks upwards. This is the biggest contraction yet, and I am starting to writhe in pain. Cliff and Gloria warble louder and louder. I think I've started to shout a bit too. Oh my God, please let this pain stop. And Gloria and Cliff too while you're at it.

'Epidural! I want an epidural!' I say to Valerie.

'OK, darling, I'll page the anaesthetist.' She gets her colleague, a spotty teenager called Rebecca, to take over, and scuttles out of the room.

It's difficult to describe in words the pain of a full-scale contraction. I feel like I'm on a street corner in a B-movie and I can hear the thud-thud of a Godzilla-type monster a few blocks away. The monster's getting nearer and nearer, louder and louder, and I know it's going to be too large for me to even think about running away from it. So I stand, like a typical B-movie woman, and start to bellow. I'm going to have to face this hideous gorgon that is double the size of a tower block, be gripped by it and have my bones crunched piecemeal in its slavering jaws.

Still no sign of Dan or Valerie or the anaesthetists. At least Cliff and Gloria have put their mikes down and are on the sofa again. Oh blimey, here we go. Now that I've experienced the level of this pain, I have started to squirm against it before it's even reached full strength.

'Try to relax,' says Rebecca.

'Oh go and read *Just Seventeen*!' I shout. I feel a grain of embarrassment. I've never met the girl before.

I notice I'm swearing quite a lot. It hasn't become really rude yet. I'm still at the 'RUDDY ADA!' and 'BLINKING NORA' stage. I'm pacing myself.

Valerie arrives with the pair of anaesthetists. They're like a little double act in green scrubs. One has perforated white clogs and the other, I notice, wears trendy green trainers. Along with foul language, details are increasingly my only defence. I'm worried that if they spend that much time shopping, their spinal tapping might be a bit rusty.

Between contractions, Valerie's latexed hand is rummaging around my interior again.

'How is it down there?' I shout. 'Still something resembling the genitals I once knew or have we gone Eurotunnel yet?'

'You're about five centimetres dilated,' she tells me.

'How long to go?' I plead.

'Could be a few hours,' she says sanguinely.

I'm sure I see a flicker of a smile on Rebecca's face as she leaves the room. Probably off for a quick alcopop or something.

The anaesthetists are called Charlie and Simon and they set to work preparing their little box of tricks. An epidural is basically a mega painkiller injected into your spinal fluid. When Stella mentioned spinal tap during our classes, Dan had momentarily sat up. I can't help but think that if men gave birth there would be thousands of laboratories set up all over the globe, dedicated night and day to coming up with new ways of easing the pain of childbirth.

Charlie looks at me, slightly confused. I can feel another contraction starting to brew.

'Have I met you before?' he says, pulling out the largest needle I've ever seen from its case.

'NUTS!' I bellow as the contraction starts to bite.

'Now you're going to have to keep extremely still for about two minutes,' says Simon, who's tinkering around with my back, preparing the area for the jab.

'STILL? STILL? I CAN'T KEEP RUDDY BLINKING STILL!'

'I really do know her,' I hear Charlie whispering to Valerie confidentially. 'It's on the tip of my tongue.'

The contraction subsides and Simon tries to get the needle into my spine. Dan arrives, winks at me, and immediately looks wary of these two whipper-snapper drugs dealers tinkering around with his wife.

'What's going on?' he says brusquely.

'Epidural,' I snap, as Dan comes to kiss me. 'AND KEEP AWAY FROM ME!'

Simon is having difficulties getting the needle in.

'You're going to have to keep really, really still, I'm afraid.'

The pain is making me squirm and writhe against my better judgement. Gloria's waving goodbye to all and sundry in her *Open House*. Tomorrow Leo Sayer will be dropping in. At this rate I'll still be here to see him. This is interminable. This is agony.

'I simply can't get into the spine with you moving around like this.'

'Anything I can do?' says Dan, involuntarily exercising his male practical gene. I don't think roofing skills really qualify him for this kind of precision work.

'What area do you live in?' says Charlie, still trying to place me.

Dan's jaw is twitching. I can see that he has taken against Charlie, and if he weren't on crutches might even try and floor him.

'OK, I've done what I can but I don't know if it's going to be one hundred per cent effective,' announces Simon.

I simply don't care any more. Strip me, wire me up to more machinery, pierce me with crochet hooks, parade my front bottom to half the hospital staff. I don't care. I am receding into my own groove of pain now and nobody can get me out of it. I want my mum. I want some crack. I don't know what I want.

I'm just about to start riding up another hill on the big dipper when Charlie clicks his fingers and smiles, all pleased with himself.

'You're on TV ... I knew I'd seen you before. With that other girl. My girlfriend quite likes you. Don't suppose you'd mind leaving an autograph for her? "To Gill" would be great. After all this is over, obviously.'

Dan is looking ominously like he's going to swing his crutch over Charlie's head, but luckily Charlie and Simon take their leave before there is unnecessary violence.

'ROGER ME TILL KINGDOM COME BUT MY GOSH THAT'S PAINFUL!'

I'll soon be swearing at full tilt with nothing in reserve.

Dan clumsily rams the gas and air mouthpiece into my gob again, and it clanks uncomfortably around my jaw. My fist lashes out and catches him full in the eye. God. The contact of my bony knuckle on his fleshy face feels good.

'HOW MUCH MORE OF THIS IS THERE?' I shout out to Valerie, as poor Dan reels backwards into a chair, clutching his eye. At least it'll stop him winking.

'Could be a while yet,' says Valerie uselessly. 'You must try to relax. Hopefully the epidural will start to take effect.'

I'm amazed when Dan tells me that it's half past three. I've been in this dungeon of pain for nearly four hours! When can I start pushing for goodness' sake? Where's the baby amidst this carnival? I go to all this trouble and the guest of honour can't even be bothered to show up. How rude is that?

Valerie has the gall to start humming to herself. She sings in a nice, relaxed way. It's a show tune and clearly one she knows and likes. That's right, Valerie, you just chill out while I'm screaming like an elephant having its testes removed.

I'm beginning to feel a numbness creeping down my left leg.

'I CAN'T FEEL MY LEFT LEG!' I scream at Valerie, who just won't stop humming.

'That sometimes happens with the epidural, darling.'

'GREAT! SO I'M GOING TO END UP LIKE DOUGLAS BLOODY BADER, AM I?'

Dan is still nursing his eye and looks pretty fed up. He comes over again and tries to stroke my hair.

From somewhere far away I'm aware of hearing the sounds of a medieval farmyard. There's a bull mooing loudly in a field over yonder. The flicker of a smile crosses Dan's face. I suddenly realise that it's me making that bellowing noise. How extraordinary. The thing is it really does help with the pain. The contractions are coming pretty much one on top of the other. It's impossible to say where one finishes and the next starts. I lose all sense of time or place, I just want to bellow like an old moo-cow.

'I NEED TO POO!' I scream at Valerie.

She looks knowingly at Dan.

'She's ready to start pushing,' she tells him.

Valerie suddenly looks me in the eye, and from very close up almost shouts in my face: 'You are going to get this baby out. I want you to push down in your bottom next time you feel a contraction.'

'CAN'T. TOO TIRED.'

'You will push. Chin down. Not from the throat. A big deep push from your bottom.'

And somehow that is what starts happening. I start to push and bellow at the same time.

It's dark outside.

Dan has taken up pole position and looks up into my body like an earnest chimney sweep. I don't think even Lionel Richie's going to do much for us after this.

'I can see the head!' shouts Dan, his eyes suddenly full of tears.

I carry on pushing and I'm pleased to report, the Vanessa Redgrave breathing actually starts to come into play here, and of its own accord! How extraordinary. Bellowing, gasping, pumping, just like in films!

'Now we need a big one! Come on, Melanie!'

'IT'S MEL!' I grunt.

I've always hated being called by my full name and even in these circumstances I will not stand for it.

I think of my Lithuanian forefathers holed up in some bloody thirteenth-century battle. I think of their strong horses and their big swords. I give it some Lithuanian-style pushing. This is for them. Here we go.

'BWAAAAAAAARRRGGGGGGGGGGHHHHHHHH.' That's a noise that the Royal Shakespeare Company would be proud of.

Dan goes a mysterious shade of blue, comes away from his crutches and falls backwards.

I'm aware of a large fish sliding out of my body. And something else very bizarre has happened. There is suddenly no more pain. Nothing. I look down below and see a white fish-like creature covered in blood and gunk, with plastered down hair and a funny creased little face.

'She's a girl!' I say to Dan. 'Look, we've got a girl!'

Dan's mouth is still open. He looks at our daughter, who I'm pleased to say is taking a leaf out of her mother's book and has started bellowing for Britain. Dan is still speechless and blue.

'Can I have a cup of strong tea, please? And four slices of toast. White with lots of butter?'

I know this probably sounds like the biggest cliché in the book, but she is the most beautiful girl I've ever seen in my entire life. Ava Gardner, step aside. Raquel Welch, you're a moose. This little angel can knock you off the catwalk any day.

Dan's turning a healthy pink again, thank goodness, and Valerie busies herself with a bit of stitching, which, strangely enough, I don't even feel. She could hack off a foot and I simply wouldn't notice, I'm in serious adrenaline heaven.

Dan and I start to crow over her.

'She looks like your dad,' says Dan.

'I love her froggy legs.'

'I love her wrinkly wrists.'

The room may be plain, surgical and unmemorable, but right now it feels like the most expensive important suite in the grandest hotel in the world and the toast might as well have beluga caviar on it.

'I bought one of those Baby on Board stickers,' says Dan.

'Oh, good idea!' I say.

Our journey has begun. I can't imagine life without her now. I feel very warmly to my previous life, but I don't want to go back there ever. Not while she's here.